HEART HEALTHY LIFESTYLE

A holistic mind, body, and soul approach to living a Heart Healthy Lifestyle

By

NIK NIKAM, M.D.

Author of *Stressless Mind & Priceless Body*

HEART HEALTHY LIFESTYLE

Senior Editor: Marta Tanrikulu
Assistant Editor: Navin Nikam, M.D.
Cover Graphics: Nik Nikam, M.D.

Nikam, Nik
Heart-Healthy Lifestyle
A mind, body, and soul approach to living a Heart Healthy Lifestyle

First Printing: March 2010

Publication Date: March 30, 2010
EAN13: 9780984412808
Language: English

SUGAR LAND HEART CENTER
16659 Southwest FWY 361
Sugar Land, TX 77479
www.sugarlandheartcenter.com.

Printed in the United States of America

HEART HEALTHY LIFESTYLE

"Concepts are a dime a dozen and those who practice them are priceless"

With Best Wishes

To_____

_____

NIK NIKAM, M.D.

Heart Healthy Living is a life transforming phenomenon. Many of my patients who have had a heart attack or a heart surgery welcome this concept. Why not live a Heart Healthy Lifestyle now, so your family and you may enjoy years of health & happiness.

Dedicated

to thousands of my patients, who challenged me with provocative questions, energized me to seek answers beyond the cardiology confines, inspired me to provide a more humanistic and holistic approach to managing their problems, and encouraged me to treat them with humility and dignity.

"Hi, Shan, how are doing? I asked.

"Hi, Dr. Nik. I'm having chest pain," he replied.

"How old are you?

"I am only 38."

"What kind of work do you do?" I asked.

"Software engineer."

"High blood pressure?" I asked.

"Yes."

"Diabetes?" I questioned.

"Yes."

"High cholesterol?

"You bet," he said.

"Family history? I asked.

"I have no family," he replied, "I take that back. I have a wife and three young kids."

"Smoking, drinking, and cursing?" I asked.

"All of the above." He smiled.

"Shan, then your wife needs a copy of my book." I smiled.

"What book?" he said.

"Heart Healthy Lifestyle." I waited for his response.

"Dr. Nik, she isn't your patient. I'm your patient. You should be talking to me." He laughed.

"Shan, I am talking to you. She needs some guidance in re-engineering your Heart Healthy Lifestyle! Besides, she is your boss."

"No! Not again! Let's not go there. You know what? I think my chest pain is back. Dr. Nik, I think I need that book, now!"

Table of Contents

Table of Contents

Table of Contents

Chapter 01

Introduction
Let the Heart Healthy Lifestyle journey begin

I am 93 Years Old, and I . . .

It was 1980. I had just moved to Houston after completing my cardiology training at Henry Ford Hospital in Detroit. It was the year when people in Detroit had bumper stickers that read, "Will the last person to leave Detroit please turn out the lights?"

I was excited about my career and profession. While I was addressing an audience in Pearland, Texas, I began, "Let's imagine for a moment that you are a proud owner of a thoroughbred race horse worth in excess of a million dollars. You have already won two major races, and now you are getting ready for that third and final race—the Kentucky Derby—to snatch the Triple Crown. You are excited, your horse is ecstatic, and all systems are ready to go. Now, you are waiting for that final pistol sound, so you can dash through the gates to the finish line. Amen!"

"Looks like we got a gambler here," yelled an elderly gentleman from the back.

"Let me pause here for a moment and ask you a couple of questions: How many of you would let this horse overindulge in eating, drinking, smoking, cursing, and dancing till three o'clock in the morning to heavy-metal rock or hip-hop music?"

A deafening silence swept the auditorium.

"Of course, you are not going to do that," I continued. "That is a one million dollar investment. Instead, you are going to hire the best veterinarian in the country to make sure that your horse is maintained in optimal health. You are going to employ the best equestrian chef in the country to provide your horse the most balanced diet possible. And you are going to hire the best stallion trainer to coach the horse in such a manner that it will win the Triple Crown, even if it means by the length of its nose at the finish line—would you not?

The expressions on the audience's faces reflected, "So what?"

I have been a speaker for many years, and I knew silence is deadly. Since it was my job to keep the momentum going, I continued, "What about you? Do you realize that undoubtedly you are racing through life in what God gave you—*a billion dollar body*? Do you think you take care of yourself as well as you would a one-million-dollar horse?"

Silence again. This time the audience looked at me like I was crazy.

"Probably not!" I continued, "That is why I am going to give you a prescription for a Heart Healthy Lifestyle. Yes, indeed you do need a prescription for a Heart Healthy Lifestyle!"

I finally paused here, thinking that I would get some applause from the audience. Again the room was quiet, lifeless except for a few sardonic giggles, which were abruptly interrupted by a 93-year-old lady, Mrs. Johnson, who stood up from the end of the hall.

"Young man," she began, "I don't know why you have come here to preach us. I am 93 years young. I am healthier than that creepy million-dollar horse you are trying to sell me. And I certainly don't need a prescription from a teenager like you."

No sooner did she finish her speech than her nursing-home colleagues rose with thunderous applause and a standing ovation—for her.

I was really astonished. Not only had she evidently lived the secrets of a Heart Healthy Lifestyle, but also she knew persuasive public speaking to impact her audience, something I had failed to do that morning.

Well, I did not lose heart, yet. As a speaker, I had bombed many times in the past and recovered before the audience could feel my agony. I was not ready to give up. Instead, I joined the audience in applause and continued, "Well ma'am, I agree with you 100 percent that you don't need a prescription. But, in reality, I only presented this story to see how many of you were awake at the beginning of my presentation."

"I am not finished yet," she shot back. "Why don't you go back to school and get a medical degree before you start selling prescriptions to old folks!"

That day, as I was driving back, I intensely pondered on the interaction I had with that wonderful 93-year-young (not old) lady. I realized I was preaching to the choir. These people had already lived long, useful lives. I wondered if I should go back to school again and research the true meaning of a Heart Healthy Lifestyle.

The fact that her words, even to this day, still reverberate in my mind and heart is a testament to the validity of her statement and conviction. Then, I recognized that I should actually be addressing the people who were just at the dawn of their adult life, those in their teens, twenties, thirties, or forties. I should be advising those who were already overindulging in eating, drinking, smoking, cursing, and practicing unhealthy lifestyles.

Hello, I'm Dr. Nik Nikam. Thanks for reading my book, "Heart Healthy Lifestyle." This book is designed to provide you with more than 25 years of pearls and wisdom that I have learned from my patients on a Heart Healthy Lifestyle.

In the past, I had given numerous health-related presentations with little or no effect on the seminar-attendees' lifestyles. Even at my office, my efforts to educate my patients on a Heart Healthy Lifestyle had a marginal impact, with the exception of those people who'd had a major heart attack or heart surgery. Even those people who adhered to my advice for a few months eventually slipped back into their routine lifestyle.

As I analyzed the deficiencies in my past techniques, I realized that my recommendations for a Heart Healthy Lifestyle were grossly inadequate. When a person signs up for a language, art, or music class, he is provided with one-on-one coaching, textbooks, reading material, homework, classroom training, internet sources and a library of information to sharpen his knowledge and accelerate his learning skills.

But, what do we offer those who entrust their hearts to us? We offer them a pocket full of pills and say, "Eat less fat and cholesterol, lose weight, exercise, and I will see you in three months; that will be $250, John!" With that type of advice, what are the chances of you seeing a noticeable change in your weight or cholesterol level? If a similar amount of instruction was given to school students, I wonder how many of them would even get a passing grade.

An exceptionally good music teacher is someone who is accomplished in her own musical talents. A healthcare professional cannot preach what he himself does not practice. In order to practice anything lifelong, those guiding principles must become second nature to you. Therefore, I felt I must design a system that I can make my lifestyle. So, I started practicing the same principles to get first-hand experience at a Heart Healthy Lifestyle. I will admit it was not easy. I realized that preaching cardiology was a piece of cake compared to practicing it on myself.

That inspired me to take a second look at the latest medical literature on a Heart Healthy Lifestyle. I spent countless hours burning the candle at both ends just trying to weed out useless commercial information, non-practical solutions, and unconventional alternatives labeled as natural or wholesome. While some books covered weight control highlighting only carbs, proteins, or fats, others only emphasized exercise, showing a herd of young body builders as models. A Heart Healthy Lifestyle is more than just losing weight or toning the oblique muscles, which most people fail to appreciate. It also addresses management of stratosphere-piercing stress levels and sky-high cholesterol levels.

After extracting the most pertinent information from the vast medical sources, I started publishing a series of easy-to-follow life-transforming articles for my patients.

We decorated our waiting room with these articles. Ironically, they were disappearing regularly from the binders, and we happily refilled them.

As I gathered more and more useful information, my 20-page handout expanded to more than 300 pages. Then it became a problem for us to reproduce those articles on our copy machine. That inspired me to write this book, so each person could have a comprehensive lifetime guide for the future.

Conversation With Kelly

The other day I was quietly making rounds in the hospital, seeing my patients, when my old friend Kelly and her cronies trapped me in the nurses' station.

"You look a little thin, Dr. Nik," Kelly smirked. "What's the matter, business isn't good?"

Let me tell you something about nurse Kelly. She is not just an ordinary nurse. I have known her for over 20 years. Not only is she sharp of mind, but also sharp of tongue. And, she assumes absolute interrogation authority over me concerning everything from patient care to my vital statistics, including belt size.

"I guess your kids are still on your payroll, and you are on a financial diet," she continued.

"What? Am I on the witness stand? You sound like a plaintiff's lawyer. Any more questions Miss—Your Honor?" I bantered back.

"Yes, Dr. Nik. As a matter of fact, we want to know if you are on a diet." They chuckled.

"No, but I have been busy with my upcoming book."

"Really! What is it called?"

"Heart Healthy Lifestyle," I said.

"I should have guessed. You are too kind-hearted to write thriller mystery novels." She smiled.

"Well, I have to get back to my work."

"No, you are not going to get off the hook so easily," shouted the cronies. "We want to know what is going to be in your book."

"It is about a Heart Healthy Lifestyle. Why don't you come to my office and read the whole book?"

"If you can't convince me in a few minutes what your book is about, there is no reason for me to come to your office and waste my time."

"Does this book have a holistic approach?" asked Kelly.

"Well, Kelly, this book deals with mind, body and soul. And, more importantly, it addresses common cardiovascular issues that we come across at all ages. I talk about chest pain in young children and elderly adults with pacemakers. I talk about the development of heart failure or peripheral arterial disease that can cause mini-strokes or problems in the legs. In the first section, I address diet-related topics, since what we eat determines our composition now and in the future."

"Then?" She asked.

"It deals with topics that are dedicated to the risk factors for heart disease and how people can modify them. Next, I address subjects that pertain to the mind and soul. Finally, I talk about preventive medicine, where many topics are covered that deal with minimizing complications related to heart disease."

"Sounds like a comprehensive approach to a Heart Healthy Lifestyle," she said, "Let's talk about diet. What kind of advice do you have for your readers?"

"This book covers in depth the role of carbohydrates and fats in the body with reference to weight gain and weight control. . ."

"Are you going to tell readers to count calories?" Kelly asked.

"Of course calorie counts are important. I will teach them how to count calories, no matter what ethnic background they come from. I cover the calorie counts based on raw foods."

"What about a vegetarian diet?"

"I dispel the myths surrounding the vegetarian diets. Not all vegetarian diets are safe. You will find out when you read that chapter."

"That's interesting." She said. "I guess you are going to talk about vegetables."

"You can eat lots of celery and lettuce, and not have to worry much about calories," I said.

"Do you recommend certain vegetables?" She asked.

"Yes, I recommend leafy vegetables. I also recommend fresh

fruits or fruit drinks. I talk about the fruits and vegetables that are high in antioxidants."

"Do I need a degree in nutrition to master your book?"

"That is the beauty of this book. I clearly explain how to count calories in your daily foods, how to control your calorie intake. I have also provided useful tips for selecting healthy breakfast, lunch and dinner menus. There is no ready-made meal that you have to buy to stay healthy. I just provide the knowledge that you can translate into any ethnic food groups and make the right choices."

"Dr. Nik, did you know the Mediterranean diet and the omega-3s are a hot topic now?"

"I have been quite interested in the value of omega-3s for several years. I take fish and flaxseed oil capsules, which contain omega-3s. Kelly, did you know that our regular diet contains less than 1% of the omega-3s we should be getting in our diet? You will learn a lot about the role of omega-3s in the body and many of their benefits.

"Do you believe in a high fiber diet?"

"Yes, I do. Fiber is not only important in our daily diet, but also has cholesterol lowering properties. Benecol has more soluble fiber that is known to bring down cholesterol levels. Once you read this chapter on fiber, you will be more friendly to your salads and fibers."

"What about drinks?"

"Just say no!" I stressed.

"I mean soft drinks."

"Ditto!"

"Are you serious?" she asked.

"Really, I thought you were referring to alcohol. If it is alcohol, I would recommend red wine. Soft drinks have empty calories and caffeine. Water is the best drink, and you need plenty of it. I have several chapters that cover fluids, drinks, and caffeine."

"As a cardiologist, you must be selling antioxidants to your patients," she said.

"I don't sell any pills to my patients. I do believe in antioxidants. They are supposed to reduce cell damage, protect cell integrity and preserve youth."

"Do you have some samples?"

"You can get most antioxidants from dark leafy vegetables and highly pigmented fruits and berries. If you read up on this topic in the book, you will also get a list of foods that can, perhaps, help you preserve your youth also."

"Okay. How are people supposed to choose breakfast, lunch, and dinner menus? Do you have hundreds of recipes like most diet books do?"

"First of all, I do not believe in recipes. I do not like to cook recipes based on a book and expect the food to taste as good as it does in the chef's kitchen. I provide the basic heart healthy choice and let people use that to make a combination of foods they like and enjoy. It is like teaching a man how to fish rather than giving him a fish. You will be delighted to read the chapter on Everyday Dinner."

"What else you are going to have in your book?" Kelly continued.

"Next, I address risk factor modification—what I call 'tune up your body!'"

"What are they going to learn here?" Kelly asked.

"I describe the structure of the human heart as an engineering marvel. I compare the structure and function of the heart based on many engineering principles, from structural to software."

"I thought you were a cardiologist!"

"Kelly, in reality, many heart functions are based on engineering principles that deal with fluid movements, valves, friction and resistance. In fact, blood pressure is based on blood flow and resistance."

"Aren't you getting too technical?" Kelly asked. "How about a simple thing like chest pain?"

"Yes, Boss! I have a chapter on chest pain alone, where we explore many different causes of chest pains and help people understand that not all chest pains are from the heart. But, it is of utmost importance to identify pains that are related to heart disease and treat them in an expeditious manner," I said.

"You are right, Dr. Nik. We see many people in the hospital with chest pain who turn out to have no heart disease and then, time and again we miss persons with a real heart problem. What next?"

"Then, I talk about cholesterol, which is the number one risk factor for heart disease. I also provide a list of 22 ways to lower cholesterol naturally."

"I think I need a cigarette break." She sighed while yawning.

"Hold it, miss, what did you say?" I asked.

"I said, I need a cigarette break."

"No, you don't. You need to read the chapter on smoking before you light another cigarette," I said.

"You don't have a chapter on exercise?"

"Exercise must be an integral part of a Heart Healthy Lifestyle. Running your fingers through the laptop keyboard or your favorite dessert is not considered exercise," I said.

"Then what is considered exercise?" she asked.

"There is a chapter covering stretching, aerobic, and strengthening exercises to improve your physical fitness, cardiac fitness, and appearance."

"What about weight control?"

"It is interesting that you ask about weight control. Houston was known as the fattest city in America. Once, when I was addressing fifth grade children, I noticed that 40% of the kids were overweight. Houston, we've got a problem! And, I have a fat chapter on weight control."

"I knew, sooner or later, you were going to talk about it."

"I have a very simple approach, where I explain why and how people accumulate weight and what steps they need to take to maintain their weight," I said.

"That's it. You are not going to tell me more about weight control."

"Kelly, it is not a diet plan with severe restriction of carbs, fats, or excess protein. It is about developing life transforming habits."

"Well, that is beyond me, what else do you have? Dr. Nik, most people would want to know something about a heart attack, and what they need to do, when and if they get one?" Kelly stressed.

"Kelly, now you sound like a smart nurse taking. You have been smart all along. Otherwise, I would have been able to talk to myself this long. You know, time is heart muscle. The sooner people get to the hospital, the greater are the chances of saving their heart muscle.

I explain in detail what people need to focus on when they think they are having a heart attack."

"Dr. Nik, I have noticed that people who are admitted with chest pain routinely use tranquilizers."

"Kelly, you see, heart disease is very complex and perplexing."

"How?"

"Heart disease plays havoc on many other systems that we need to understand to live a meaningful life with heart disease or to help someone with heart disease in the family."

"I think you make a lot of sense. I have seen some doctors walking in and out of a heart attack patient's room not even looking at the patient or listening to his concerns."

"Whenever someone has heart disease, anxiety, panic attacks, stress, lack of sleep, depression, and many other emotional problems complicate the issue."

"I'm glad you're addressing those points, which no one pays attention to. Patients deserve better medical care."

"I go beyond those common issues, and expand on the importance of sound sleep, music and health, and having a sense of humor. We need to have a balanced life to get through tremendous challenges placed on our mind, body and soul on a daily basis."

"I didn't think you were a shrink. Where did you learn the relationship between heart and anxiety, stress, depression, music and humor?"

"When you deal with heart patients for 25 years, they are going to teach you a lot more than any textbook can teach."

"Does that mean that you have weathered and wrinkled during these past 25 years?"

"Excuse me, Miss!"

"It is a joke, Dr. Nik! You said we need to have a sense of humor!" she said.

"Ah, ha! You got me there." I surrendered.

"You know what you should focus on? The buzz word today is 'Preventive Medicine.' People face many complications related to their heart disease, because they don't get preventive care."

"I thought I was the only one who was overdosed on the healthcare bill. Actually, there are many complications that can be prevented with timely treatment of conditions associated with heat and heart disease."

"Did you know, a friend of mine had a baby, and she was told that she had heart failure? She is only 23 years old. I was really surprised."

"Kelly, you are right. Some people can develop heart failure after pregnancy. Therefore, I have devoted an entire chapter to pregnancy and heart disease. Women experience many symptoms, most of which are harmless. Some of them require utmost attention. While we are on the topic of women, I also have included a chapter on women and heart disease. Interestingly, women after menopause have the same risk of getting heart disease as men."

"What are looking at me for? I am nowhere close to menopause."

"That is the point. Women need to pay attention to the risk factors as much as men do, once they pass age 30 or 40. I have a chapter on women and osteoporosis."

"Nik, these are very important issues to women. I am glad you're addressing women's issues. Now I have to change my perception of you."

"Most people are concerned about high blood pressure. I also talk about low blood pressure. I talk about how to recognize low blood pressure and treat it with simple remedies."

"What about high blood pressure?" she asked.

"You know that high blood pressure is one of the major risk factors for heart disease. Controlling blood pressure will not only reduce the risk of heart disease, but also will dramatically reduce the risk of stroke. You will be interested in reading about high blood pressure treatment along with knowing about low blood pressure, which is rarely talked about."

"Diabetes runs in my family. I am afraid that it's only a matter of time before I will feel the symptoms of diabetes." Kelly sounded worried.

"I am glad you are worried about it now, and not after you've developed many complications. Diabetes is a major risk factor for heart disease, and when treated aggressively, you can reduce the damage to multiple organs such as heart, kidneys, and blood vessels," I said.

"Dr. Nik, that reminds me of a patient who had a TIA or mini-stroke in her forties. How could that be possible?"

"You are talking about a peripheral arterial disease that can develop in people with multiple risk factors and especially in people with diabetes. I discuss arterial disease in the legs, the carotids and the brain. I also discuss the causes of transient ischemic attack (TIA) or mini-stroke."

"While we are on the subject of stroke, what about blood thinners? They are a real problem. If it is less than what is needed, it may not protect against clot formation, and when there is too much in the blood, people have an increased risk of bleeding," Kelly said.

"That is very true. As a nurse, you can appreciate the double-edged sword nature of blood thinners. I have devoted an entire chapter to this topic to help people understand the importance of blood thinners, their uses, dangers, and most importantly, how they can minimize such dangers," I said.

"Is it possible to prevent congestive heart failure altogether?" Kelly asked.

"I am really impressed with your curiosity. As much as we have understood heart disease, we have a lot to learn about congestive heart failure. It seems like most heart patients are eventually headed in that direction. The most important point from a patient perspective is to see how they can monitor their symptoms, minimize events that worsen heat failure, take their medicines, and avoid hospital admissions. I describe what the heart failure drugs do and what surgical options are available," I said.

"Hopefully, that should alleviate a lot of their anxiety and apprehension. Dr. Nik, maybe you should include a chapter on medication errors. You know that is a very hot topic now," Kelly said.

"You must be reading my mind. Thousands of people die in the hospitals each year from meditation errors, most of which are preventable. Many people do not get the desired effects of their medicines because there are many factors which are overlooked. I cover all these aspects in one chapter and make recommendations on how patients need to be vigilant about their medicine, and what they are getting. I also talk about why some medicines don't work."

"Dr. Nik, some patients ask me about irregular heartbeats. They want to know if they need a pacemaker. I don't know the answer. I tell them to ask their doctors," Kelly said.

"What do you mean, you don't know? You are an ICU nurse!" I chuckled, "I get your point. Atrial fibrillation is the most common rhythm problem we come across. It is an important rhythm problem, because it can cause symptoms due to rapid heartbeats, worsening heart failure, and possibly cause a stroke due to blood clot formation. I will discuss all these and much more including the indications for pacemakers and defibrillators."

"What about controversial topics like drug-coated or bare metal stents, stem cell research...?"

"In my concluding chapter on 'Innovations in Treatments,' I discuss the controversy that surrounds the debate about drug-coated stents versus bare mental stents. I stress the importance of what people need to know, since it concerns their lives. Stem cell research opens a new chapter in the treatment of heart disease. Though it is highly experimental, one day it might help us better treat patients with heart attack or heart failure. I also talk about the new test that might identify who is at a risk of developing a heart disease, when conventional tests are normal."

"Dr. Nik, that is amazing! With that amount of information packed in this little book, where does anyone start?"

"Like any other project we venture into in life, we must begin with a vision in our mind. We need to have a vision of what a Heart Healthy Lifestyle is. So, they need to proceed to the next step, 'From a Vision to a Virtual Reality, '" I said.

"I've got to go. My patient is calling. Nice talking to you, Dr. Nik. When you do finish your book, don't forget my free copy!" Kelly said.

Notes:

Chapter 02

From a Vision to a Reality

"Begin with the end in mind."
Steven Covey

Where Are You Today?

Since you can't reach a destination that you don't already have in mind, or come back from a place you've never been, you need to define a vision of a Heart Healthy Lifestyle before you can get there. Once you have defined your current situation, you need to get motivated, map the new coordinates, and take the first step toward a Heart Healthy Lifestyle. As you voyage through fresh and unfamiliar terrain, you need a clear knowledge of the new challenges that you are likely to encounter. Once you reach your destination, you still need unrelenting enthusiasm and dedication to maintain your Heart Healthy Lifestyle.

"What makes up a Heart Healthy Lifestyle?" you may wonder.

The first incidence of coronary heart disease was referenced in the medical literature in 1903. In a span of just over one hundred years, we have learned more about heart disease than what we learned in the past thousand years. Now we know that high cholesterol, smoking, high blood pressure, obesity, and diabetes increase the incidence of heart disease. More importantly, we also have learned that reducing or eliminating these risk factors can dramatically reduce the risk of heart disease and its complications. People can live longer and enjoy better lives by following a Heart Healthy Lifestyle.

Here is my definition of a Heart Healthy Lifestyle

	Items
	Cholesterol < 200 mg%
	LDL (bad cholesterol) < 80 mg%
	HDL (good cholesterol) > 40 mg%
	Triglycerides < 150 mg%
	Smoke-free lifestyle
	Diabetes control (HgA1c < 7.0)
	Blood pressure control (< 130/80 mm Hg)
	Height-based body weight (BMI < 25)
	Routine exercise regimen
	Practice of meditation
	Social involvement
	Sense of humor
	Minimal cursing (stress level)
	Stress reduction training
	Heart healthy food choices
	Realistic expectations
	Living the Heart Healthy Lifestyle

In a real sense, the Heart Healthy Lifestyle is more than just a definition or a destination. It is a lifelong transformation and a state of well-being. Presently, we may be unable to cure diabetes and high blood pressure, or genetic problems. However, we certainly can reduce our heart disease risk by controlling many risk factors and eliminating others, while cultivating a few fresh habits along the way.

Inventory: First, you need a checkup from the toes up. If you are over 40 or have a family history of heart disease, get a comprehensive medical examination to determine your general health and assess your heart disease risk. Set aside a weekend to complete your Heart Healthy Lifestyle Checklist. Gather information on your weight, blood pressure readings, and blood sugar and cholesterol levels. Take an inventory of your eating habits for a week, and follow the chart below to record your choices. Completing the following checklist will serve as the starting point on your Heart Healthy lifestyle journey.

Heart Healthy Lifestyle Checklist

Items	Current	Vision
Cholesterol < 200 mg%		
LDL (bad cholesterol) < 80 mg%		
HDL (good cholesterol) > 40 mg%		
Triglycerides < 150 mg%		
Smoke-free lifestyle		
Diabetes control (HgA1c < 7.0)		
Blood pressure control (< 130/80 mm Hg)		
Height-based body weight (BMI < 25)		
Routine exercise regimen: Yes/No		
Practice of meditation: Yes/No		
Social involvement: Yes/No		
Sense of humor: Yes/No		
Cursing (stress level): Yes/No		
Stress reduction training: Yes/No		
Heart healthy food choices: Yes/No		
Realistic expectations: Yes/No		
Living the Heart Healthy Lifestyle: Yes/No		

Get your electrolytes checked, since a calorie-restrictive diet can alter them. Thyroid hormone is intricately involved in your over-all metabolism. Low thyroid hormone levels promote water retention and interfere with muscle function, while high thyroid hormone levels increase metabolism, leading to weight and muscle loss. If you are over 40, consider an electrocardiogram and a stress test before you enroll in a regular exercise program. Keep copies of your medical tests so that you can compare them in the future and track your progress.

Road Map to Your Vision

Motivation: Motivation is like the spark plug that ignites your passion for a Heart Healthy Lifestyle. Remember that one dose of motivation is not adequate. Every time you wander off course, you need another dose of extra energy to steer you back on course. A regular follow-up with your physician could provide you with that enduring motivation to live a Heart Healthy Lifestyle.

Practice: If you ask a realtor what is the most important thing to consider when buying property, you will hear "location, location, location." When it comes to rebuilding your body and cultivating a Heart Healthy lifestyle, I will say, "practice, practice, practice." First, practice the habits outlined in the Heart Healthy Lifestyle Checklist. Second, practice. It takes time to see results. You cannot go from a cholesterol level of 300 mg% to 200 mg% in ten days. Finally, practice persistence. Since the results can be slow to come and difficult to perceive, you are likely to give up on certain heart healthy habits and seek the path of least resistance. Therefore, you have to triumph over your temptations and weaknesses.

Strategy: When you desire a positive, decisive change in your lifestyle, you should have a multidimensional approach for a Heart Healthy Lifestyle. You should address your eating, drinking, smoking, cursing, and sedentary lifestyle habits all at the same time. By doing so, you will begin to see some positive changes, which will fuel your enthusiasm further to cultivate more and more Heart

Healthy Lifestyle habits.

"That's easier said than done," you may say.

You may be right. Yet, cultivating a Heart Healthy Lifestyle is much easier than experiencing a major heart attack while lying in the intensive care unit in a foreign land with your life hanging by IV fluids.

I have heard many people in intensive care and cardiac surgery units saying, "I was fixing to go on this diet program, and then this heart attack came along," or "As soon as I get out of hospital, I am going to change my entire lifestyle." Once, an inspirational speaker said, "Fear is one of the greatest motivators for mankind." I can attest to the validity of his sentiment by recalling the expressions of my heart patients while lying in the intensive care units after having suffered heart attacks, rushing to embark on a Heart Healthy Lifestyle program the moment someone mentions the word, **heart attack**.

The best time to change your lifestyle is now, before you get a heart attack.

Easy bits to chew: Break down your long-term vision into smaller and more manageable goals. Losing 25 pounds in six months may seem like an impossible task. However, when you break it down, it translates into less than one pound per week. Practically speaking, it should be within anyone's reach to lose a pound a week. Once you repeat the same process week after week for several weeks, losing weight becomes easier and easier, as it brings you within striking distance of a 25-pound weight-loss goal.

Obstacles: Here are some common excuses I have heard over the years:

- But I don't have time.
- Doc, it is too hard. I cannot live like that.
- I am the CEO of seven companies, and I don't have the time.
- I travel a lot, and I have a lot of business meetings.

My response to such comments is usually:

- Do you spend time in front of a TV?
- Do you take time to have a drink?
- Do you have time to curse?
- Do you waste 30 to 60 minutes a day waiting for clients or papers?

In reality, it takes less time a day than a 30-minute TV show to nurture a Heart Healthy lifestyle.

If you were the CEO of seven companies and cultivated an unhealthy business practice, would you still be in business? If you have the time to sketch, prioritize, and execute your business plans, why don't you have time for an excellent Heart Healthy Lifestyle agenda for your body? Is your business more vital than your body? What happens when your body fails? Other than your immediate family, would anyone care? Anyone can replace you as the next CEO of your company. But can anyone replace your body? Your life?

There are different types of people. Some glorify the past with comments such as, "Those were the good old days! It's all over now." Then there are others who spend so much time in planning that they never start anything. They are just going from one plan to the other. However, there are some who are willing to risk learning new heart healthy habits for some future benefit. Go ahead—take the challenge and the risk. It might save you from a heart attack.

Heart Healthy Lifestyle Practice List

1	Reduce your calorie intake to less than _____/day (1200 to 1800) for weight loss.
2	Reduce carbohydrate intake to 200 to 800 calories, 50 to 200 grams/day for weight loss.
3	Keep fat intake to less than 20% to 30% of total calories (240 to 540 calories), or 26 to 60 grams/day.
4	Minimize intake of solid fats, sweets, butter, and lard.
5	Consume less than 15% to 25% of total calories (180 to 300) as protein, or 45 to 100 grams/day.
6	Look for skim milk instead of regular, 2% or 1% milk.
7	Select fiber-rich products: Fiber One, All-Bran, Raisin Bran, or Kashi.
8	Take 1 tbsp of Bene-fiber with 2 to 3 glasses of water (lowers cholesterol level).
9	Consider a glass (3.5 oz) of red wine per day (it is high in antioxidants, reduces heart-disease risk).
10	Consume 2 to 3 fish oil capsules twice a day (omega-3s reduce heart disease risk).
11	Take one flaxseed oil capsule twice daily (omega-3s reduce heart disease risk).
12	Consider 500 mg of niacin 1 to 3 times per day (lowers cholesterol level).
13	Exercise: Walk for 30 to 45 minutes per day or jog for 15 to 20 minutes per day. Burn at least 300 calories daily with aerobic exercise.
14	Restrict meats to less than 8 oz/day. Select chicken, turkey, lean meat, beans, peas, or veggie patties.
15	Consume fish such as salmon, mackerel, tuna, or sardines 2 to 3 times per week (omega-3s reduce heart disease risk).
16	Select salads with low-calorie dressings every day.
17	Watch a comedy channel: Get a sense of humor; it's good for the soul and nerves.
18	Downsize your belt. Never upsize your belt. Just say no.
19	Drink at least 8 glasses of water a day.
20	Take one Centrum A to Z daily.
21	Consider one aspirin tablet per day (81 or 325 mg).

Notes:

Chapter 03

Carbohydrates
On Everyone's Mind

Types of Dietary Carbohydrates

Carbohydrates are one of the major energy sources in our diet. They mostly come from plants that store solar energy in small building units called saccharides (sugars). Different saccharide forms are as follows:

Simple carbohydrates: Monosaccharides contain one saccharide unit such as glucose, fructose, or galactose. Glucose comes from table sugar, fructose comes from fruits, and galactose comes from milk.

Disaccharides, such as maltose, sucrose, and lactose, each contain two saccharide molecules. Maltose, which comes from malt syrup, contains two glucose units. Sucrose, which comes from sugar, has glucose and fructose. Lactose, found in milk, has glucose and galactose.

Oligosaccharides have five to six units of glucose or other monosaccharides. Polysaccharides contain long strings or branched chains of saccharides (like pearl beads in a necklace). Some polysaccharides such as cellulose are straight chains, whereas others such as glycogen are branched chains. Starches are polysaccharides found in cereals, beans, peas, and potatoes.

Fermentation of carbohydrates produces ethyl alcohol, which is the same alcohol found in wine and beer. Each gram of ethyl alcohol provides seven calories of energy, unlike most carbohydrates, which provide four calories.

Food sources rich in simple carbohydrates

Monosaccharides	Sources
Glucose	Fruit, honey, and corn syrup
Fructose	Fruit, honey, juices, and corn syrup
Galactose	Fruit, honey
Mannose	Pineapple, carrots, and olives

Disaccharides	Examples
Sucrose	Table sugar, maple syrup
Lactose	Milk and milk products
Maltose	Malt products and some cereals

Derivatives	Examples
Ethyl alcohol	Fermented grains
Lactic acid	Milk and milk products
Malic acid	Fruits

Complex carbohydrates: Complex carbohydrates contain polysaccharides that consist of numerous saccharide units connected.

Refined carbohydrates: They result from fiber removal from complex carbohydrates. Breaking carbohydrates into smaller saccharide units also increases their absorption rate, thus raising their glycemic index (GI), which is explained later in this chapter.

Fibers: These are large carbohydrate molecules that are resistant to the human digestive process. They can be soluble or insoluble. The soluble fibers do not directly affect digestion. They undergo bacterial fermentation in the large intestine, producing short-chain fatty acids that are absorbed in the colon. Fermentable fiber provides roughly two calories for each gram. The insoluble fibers absorb water and slow food digestion. Indigestible or insoluble fiber helps the transportation of nutrients and waste products across the intestinal tract. It also lowers pressure within the gut and promotes bowel regularity.

Food sources rich in complex carbohydrates

Digestible Complex Carbohydrates

Types	Sources
Polysaccharides	Amylose
Starch and dextrin	Grains, legumes, and vegetables
Glycogen	Meats

Partially Digestible Complex Carbohydrates

Inulin	Jerusalem artichokes, onions
Mannose	Legumes (beans, peas), called pulses
Raffinose	Sugar beets, kidney and navy beans
Stachyose	Dried beans
Pentoses	Fruits and gums

Indigestible Complex Carbohydrates (Dietary Fiber)

Cellulose	Vegetables and seeds
Hemicellulose	Vegetables and seeds
Pectin	Apple and other fruit sources

Source: Mahan, L.K. and Escott-Stump, S. Krause's Food, Nutrition & Diet Therapy, 10th ed., 2000.

Most carbohydrates come from plant sources. Most vegetable sources contain some carbohydrates. Therefore, it is important to count the invisible carbohydrate calories in foods such as starches, beans, and fruits when calculating your daily calorie intake. Carbohydrates provide your energy needs. Excess carbohydrates that are not used are converted into glycogen and stored in the liver and muscle tissues. Glycogen serves as the reserve for immediate energy needs during exercise or periods of starvation. Your body stores less than 200 grams of glycogen. Any surplus carbohydrates not stored as glycogen will be converted into fat and deposited in your fatty tissue.

Consumption of excess carbohydrates promotes insulin surges, leading to fat deposition and weight gain. The weight gain promotes insulin resistance and stimulates more insulin production, leading to hyperinsulinism (overproduction of insulin). Hyperinsulinism is one of the major problems seen in obese and diabetic people.

Although your body can burn carbohydrates, proteins, fats, and alcohol for energy, it cannot store alcohol. Therefore, it has to utilize all the energy that comes from alcohol. Normally, your body uses carbohydrates, proteins, and fats, in that order, for its energy sources. Immediately following a meal, your body has an excess carbohydrate source. However, between meals, your carbohydrate sources are low, so your body burns fat for a constant energy source. Hence, a well-balanced carbohydrate intake providing just enough energy between meals, but not so much that it turns into fat, is a vital concept in weight control. Let your body use its own fat for a continual energy source. If you plan to lose weight, do so by lowering your carbohydrate intake to less than what your body needs from meal to meal. In contrast to the Atkins diet, which recommends an unlimited fat intake, *I recommend that you let your body use its own abundant fat reserve you are trying to get rid of.* Your body knows how much fat to mobilize in a systematic fashion, as opposed to your mouth, which does not know when to stop eating.

Carbohydrates in the Body

The body stores carbohydrates in four major forms. The most important form, namely glucose, circulates in the blood to provide an instantaneous energy source. The second form, glycogen, provides energy over an extended period. The next form, fiber, makes up the structural foundation of human tissues and their support network. The final form, glycoproteins, are a combination of complex carbohydrates and proteins. These glycoproteins play an important role in carrying chemicals, hormones, and enzymes in the blood. Polysaccharides may have hundreds of thousands of monosaccharide units. Some polysaccharides such as cellulose are linear chains, whereas others such as glycogen are branched chains.

Carbohydrate Quality (Glycemic Index)

The glycemic index (GI) refers to the quality of the carbohydrates we consume. It is based on the rate at which a given carbohydrate raises your blood sugar level compared to pure glucose. Following ingestion of carbohydrate, if your blood sugar rises as quickly as it would with pure glucose, then that carbohydrate has a GI of 100. Therefore, carbohydrates with a high GI raise your blood sugar levels quickly and increase the insulin demand.

Benefits of lower GI foods: They not only raise your blood sugar gradually, compared to high GI foods, but also do not cause sudden insulin surges. Lower GI foods provide energy over a longer period than high GI foods, while also reducing hunger. Over the long term, they lessen your risk of diabetes.

Look at the chart at the end of this chapter that lists foods with lower and higher GI. This should help you to choose the right type of carbohydrates. Select foods with a GI of 50 or less.

You may have to adjust your daily eating habits to include carbohydrates with a GI of 50 or lower in your dietary routine. Reduce high GI foods such as white rice, purified flour, or white bread. It may signal a major change in your dietary culture, if not your religion! Using low GI foods will also promote overall health, since you will be eating better quality carbohydrates that your body deserves. Replace high GI carbohydrate servings with lower GI fruits and vegetables that also provide fiber, minerals, nutrients, vitamins, enzymes, flavor, and freshness without the preservatives.

Diabetics and endurance athletes have used low GI foods for years. It grabbed public attention when two diet books, *The Zone* and *Sugar Busters*, with high protein diet plans came onto the market. The authors of these books claimed that by choosing foods with low GI ratings, it was possible to achieve a rapid and steady weight loss. However, their ideas and their diets remain controversial.

The GI of individual foods will change when they are combined with other foods. Thus, it is best to mix foods that have a GI of 50 or more with salads and meat so the overall GI will be much lower.

Drawbacks of GI ratings: GI ratings are for individual foods and not for food combinations (meals or snacks). The American Diabetes Association states that the GI ratings of many foods are less accurate when the foods are eaten together at mealtimes. For example, jelly or jam has a high GI rating, but when eaten together with whole-wheat bread, your body digests the jelly and bread combination more slowly, thus reducing the final GI rating.

Fatty foods, such as chocolates, sausages, and peanuts, when mixed with carbohydrates, slow digestion. That leads to an ultimately lower GI. Yet there is a clear, statistical correlation between excess fat (low GI) consumption and obesity-related illnesses such as heart disease, diabetes, and strokes. Therefore, following a diet plan based solely on a low GI may prove to be unsafe. A more logical approach would be to combine low GI carbohydrates with vegetables, fruits, or fiber-rich products. This combination lowers the eventual GI and reduces your fat intake.

Increasing the stomach acidity with lemon juice or vinegar or citrus fruits decreases the carbohydrate absorption rate in the stomach by slowing the food-emptying rate from the stomach.

Carbohydrate Metabolism

Did you know that your blood contains less than 20 grams of glucose? It is less than the amount of carbohydrate found in a soft drink or a doughnut. Now, you wonder, what happens to the other six soft drinks that you consume daily? Well! Just look under your belt!

Excess dietary carbohydrates are stored as glycogen (up to 450 to 500 grams) in the liver and muscle. Glycogen provides energy for about 16 hours. Contrast that to the unlimited amount of energy your body can store as fat.

In extreme circumstances, a human being can survive for as long as 30 to 90 days without any food. Mahatma Gandhi proved it. Some obese people have survived over a year without food. However, I do not recommend that you starve yourself to fit your peers' image of you. In fact, trying to impress someone can be a futile contest. What happens once you impress that person? What will happen to your driving force? Cultivate a fundamental behavioral change and adopt a Heart Healthy Lifestyle.

When the blood glucose level drops, the body releases glucose from the glycogen stores in the liver or muscles to provide short-term energy. However, if the glycogen stores are low, your body generates glucose from non-carbohydrate sources, such as amino acids or fatty acids, by a process known as gluconeogenesis (new glucose formation). The pancreas produces two hormones, insulin and glucagon, that regulate the blood sugar levels. As the blood sugar (glucose) level rises, the pancreas stimulates insulin production, which transfers glucose into the liver, muscle, and fatty tissue. As the blood sugar level falls, the pancreas releases glucagon, which promotes new glucose formation.

Insulin increases glucose transfer into the liver or muscles, increases the body's absorption of amino acids, and promotes protein synthesis. However, it also promotes long-chain fatty acid synthesis (fat formation) and storage by a process known as lipogenesis. Each time you load your body with carbohydrates, you are promoting fat buildup. Therefore, the key to preventing fat buildup is to keep your carbohydrate intake matching your daily energy requirements. Excess insulin causes arterial damage. In the long run, frequent insulin surges lead to insulin resistance and hyperinsulinism (increased insulin production), due to your body's decreased ability to respond to insulin surges. Insulin resistance is commonly seen in grossly obese and diabetic people.

While insulin decreases your blood sugar level, adrenaline increases it by promoting the breakdown of glycogen in the liver and muscle tissues during stressful periods. When the blood glucose level falls below a certain critical level (60 mg%), the body stimulates adrenaline and glucagon release to maintain the blood glucose level in a narrow range between 80 to 110 mg%. If the blood glucose level continues to drop, a person can get confused or lose consciousness. A drastically low blood sugar level (hypoglycemia) can eventually lead to brain damage. A low blood sugar level often occurs during periods of vigorous exercise, fasting, excess insulin production, or alcohol consumption. This underscores the need to provide enough carbohydrates during such periods.

Ketone bodies: A much-debated topic among diet experts is the formation of ketones in the body. Ketones are produced when the body breaks down fat during prolonged exercise, periods of fasting, or starvation. Excess intake of fatty foods can also lead to excess ketone production. People on weight control programs also produce excess amounts of ketones as they mobilize their body's fat stores. Ketones are produced no matter whether you are on a very low carbohydrate diet, are starving, or are on a high protein diet. So, ketones are the result of excess fatty acids in the blood coming from dietary fat or body fat. Ketones are neither bad nor good as long as they are in reasonable limits. Surplus ketones in the blood can lead to unpleasant results such an acetone smell in the breath and acidosis (too much acid in the blood), which happens with unrestricted fat intake. In summary, you can keep your ketone levels low by reducing the total fat intake while you are on a weight control program.

How Much Carbohydrate Do You Need?

Carbohydrates contribute 50% to 80% of the calories in the present-day American diet. No wonder the Atkins diet worked for so many, especially when they were forced to reduce their total calorie intake by 60% to 70%. However, other cardiologists and I strongly disagree with Atkins unrestricted fat recommendations. Numerous studies have shown a direct correlation between increased saturated fat intake and increased heart disease incidence.

The rationale for a low carbohydrate diet does have some merit. A low carbohydrate diet forces you to cut empty calories that you do not need. However, I feel there is no need to load your system with excess fatty foods. Your body has the ability to mobilize its own fat for energy, in an orderly manner, during a low carbohydrate diet.

Ironically, most people do not need much carbohydrate to survive. Contrary to the U.S. government's dietary recommendations that 50% to 60% of your daily calories come from carbohydrates, you can survive on a diet with less than 50 grams of carbohydrates per day, which equates to 200 calories or 10% of the calories, if you are on a 2000 calorie diet. The human brain, which mainly depends on glucose for its energy, can survive on stored fatty acids during prolonged fasting or during low carbohydrate diets. The body has the ability to produce glucose using fatty acids or amino acids. Ideally, your body needs about 200 grams of carbohydrates per day (6.6 ounces of sugar or 750 calories). If you keep your carbohydrate intake to less than 200 grams per day, your body will be forced to burn fat from within. Mobilizing your own body fat will promote weight loss. If you are trying to lose weight, restrict your carbohydrate intake to less than 100 grams per day. On the other hand, if you are trying to maintain your current weight, then you can increase your carbohydrate intake up to 200 grams per day.

Try to evenly divide your daily carbohydrate allowance among meals. In other words, do not consume an entire day's carbohydrate allowance in one meal. Try to limit your carbohydrate intake to less than 30 to 40 grams per meal. This will allow your body to burn all the dietary carbohydrates for immediate energy needs.

Snacking between meals with carbohydrate rich foods is a definite way to spoil your weight loss program. As long as your body is getting quick and easy energy from carbohydrates, there is no need for it to take the extra effort to break down its own fat. People with low blood sugar problems may have to depend on five or six meals per day to keep up their blood sugar levels. If you have special medical needs, please consult with your physician. Even those people with low blood sugar levels may benefit from choosing low GI foods. These foods will maintain their blood sugar levels over a longer duration than foods with high GI carbohydrates. If you have a craving for snacks between meals, consider eating a low GI food (such as fruit, vegetables, or nuts). Limit your intake of foods containing purified sugar: sweets, jams, soft drinks, cakes, biscuits, or ice cream (I know, what's left?).

Carbohydrates in fruits and vegetables are actually unrefined sugars. Fresh fruits and vegetables also contain vital phytochemicals and other micronutrients that protect us against serious illnesses such as heart disease and cancer. The fiber in fruits, vegetables, and pulses also help lower your blood cholesterol level. Take into account the carbohydrate content in pulses like beans and lentils when planning your daily meals.

Among cereals, select Fiber One, All-Bran, or oatmeal that have low GI carbohydrates as well as high fiber content. Fiber helps to lower your cholesterol level. Choose whole-wheat bread instead of white bread. Select whole grain products such as whole-wheat bread, or pasta that contains the bran and germ. Ask for whole-wheat tortillas in place of white tortillas, brown rice instead of white rice, or basmati rice as a substitute for instant white rice. Replace white bread or rice with beans or lentils in your lunch or dinner.

As you exercise, your muscles first burn glucose for energy and then switch to glycogen stored in the muscle or liver. During periods of vigorous, energy-demanding activities, you can increase your carbohydrate intake to match your caloric demand. If you do not provide extra carbohydrate calories, your body will burn more fat, enhancing weight loss. Hence, exercise should get as much attention as your diet while trying to slim your waist or hips.

Endurance athletes need a carbohydrate-rich diet to maximize their muscle glycogen stores. Sucrose and glucose restore glycogen stores more rapidly than fructose or other carbohydrates. Thus, pure glucose would be the preferred carbohydrate to consume during athletic events. Following activity, starches or high-fiber carbohydrate sources are just as effective as simple sugars in restoring glycogen stores.

If you consume 30 to 40 grams of carbohydrates during a meal, they contribute 120 to 160 calories. If you walk, jog, or do any kind of exercise, you will essentially burn all those calories. That will ultimately force your body to use excess body fat to provide energy between your meals. It makes perfect sense to spend a good amount of time on a dance floor after you overindulge in a carbohydrate- or fat-rich diet at parties. Exercise burns those excess calories, makes you more energetic, and helps you to sleep better. You also can take a walk for 30 to 40 minutes following a heavy meal, which will enable you to burn most of the excess calories. Here is another plan: Engage yourself in moderately heavy exercise just before you go for a carbohydrate-rich dinner. By exercising, you burn most of the carbohydrates and deplete your body of glycogen stores so that any excess carbohydrates you eat will replenish those glycogen stores, instead of turning into fat.

Dietary Carbohydrate Sources

Sugar: Table sugar sold in the market is a carbohydrate with one glucose and one fructose unit. It has a GI of 65%, in contrast to white rice with a GI of 86%. Sugar raises your blood glucose level at a slower pace than white rice or Rice Krispies. Then why do so many people consider sugar to be bad? If you use it in moderation, it is neither bad nor good. It gets bad when you indulge in a can of soda containing an equivalent of nine teaspoons of sugar or your favorite dessert containing 40 to 50 grams of pure sugar per serving.

While sitting in a doctors' dining room, it amazes me to see some of my colleagues putting three, four, or even five teaspoons of sugar in their coffee or tea, in addition to five or six servings of Half & Half. They are not concerned about the empty calories, despite having full knowledge of the ramifications. I try not to share my views, since I am a minority in the group. Some of them say, "Man! Someone can sit and count calories all day long and then get hit by a truck or develop a cancer. You gotta enjoy while you can!" Well, I do have some recommendations for those with a sweet tooth affliction. If you are after the sweetness, consider using a sugar substitute.

Sugar substitutes: One teaspoon of Equal has the sweetness of two teaspoons of sugar, while one teaspoon of Splenda has the same sweetness as a teaspoon of sugar. If you need more than two teaspoons of sugar, opt for a sugar substitute so you can continue to enjoy your coffee or dessert. Yes, the sugar substitutes taste unusual, but after two to three weeks, you will get accustomed to it. Once your body has adjusted to the new taste, you will not miss your sugar. There are many different sugar substitutes, including Equal, Splenda, Sweet'N Low, and NutraSweet. Equal and NutraSweet contain Aspartame, which has been linked to cancer in experimental animals, though not proven to cause cancer in human beings.

Breads: Breads not only form the foundation of the diet pyramid, but also significantly contribute to our generous silhouette and contour. They are the major sources of our carbohydrate excess. They come in many shapes and sizes. We consume breads for breakfast, lunch, and dinner. Most snacks contain carbohydrates. Breads surround us whenever we sit at the dinner table.

Item	Carbs, g	Calories	Fiber, g
White bread	11-14	70	
Large bagel	75	300	
Whole-wheat bread	10	40-70	2-3
Fiber-rich tortilla	10-12	50	10

You can find them in the regular bread section of most supermarkets. Read the labels. If you look long enough, you will find a brand that has a combination similar to the one described above. You can find tortillas that have 10 to 12 grams of carbohydrates, 8 to 12 grams of fiber, and 50 calories per serving. How about that for a heart healthy choice? "Yes, but it tastes like grass," say my friends. You can easily reduce 40% to 50% of your daily calories from carbohydrates by making the right heart healthy choices. The tables at the end of this chapter provide you with a wide range of choices for low calorie carbohydrates with high fiber content.

Rice: I grew up in India eating rice products for breakfast, lunch, and dinner. Most of our snacks are made up of rice flour. Is rice bad? White rice, with a GI of 86%, raises the blood sugar level quickly and stimulates insulin production. The second major problem has to do with quantity. Since cooked rice does not come in known measures, there is a tendency among rice eaters to keep on eating until their stomach cannot accommodate any more. I know this from personal experience. The situation gets worse when your mind is preoccupied in an intellectual debate with your snobby friend at a dinner table during a weekend party. On the way home, when you tell your spouse, "Pass the antacid, please!" you know you overdosed on rice. Unfortunately, this may be repeated day after day at home and at weekend parties. First, make sure that your spouse serves you only half a cup of cooked rice per meal. If you want extra rice, you'd better have a good reason! Second, use basmati rice, which has a lower GI (58), instead of white rice (86). Next, consider having whole-wheat bread or fiber-rich tortillas in place of white rice.

Potatoes: Along with corn, they are a major carbohydrate source in the western world. Potatoes can be sliced, diced, crushed, chopped, mashed, or blended to please your palate. A potato has a GI of 85%. It raises the blood sugar level quickly. Most of the guidelines outlined for rice would also apply to potatoes as well.

Beans: *They* are an excellent source of protein. They also contain carbohydrates, in addition to salt and fiber. Whenever possible, substitute your pure carbohydrate serving with a bean serving. Refer to the chapter on proteins for complete information on beans.

Flour: Highly purified white flour has several disadvantages. It contains very small particles that increase the surface area available for the digestive juices and absorption. This increased absorptive surface raises the GI. Leavening agents such as yeasts or baking soda further increase the amount of surface area available for the digestive juices. In contrast, pasta has a lower GI because of having less surface area compared to pure white bread. Surprisingly, whole-wheat bread has the same GI as white bread. Even so, whole-wheat bread has many advantages, including higher fiber content.

Fruits: The body's ability to digest fructose, a common monosaccharide found in fruits and honey, is considerably less compared to pure glucose. Fruits do not stimulate the insulin surges seen with white rice, flour, or pasta. Therefore, supplying your carbohydrates in the form of fruits makes sense. Fruits provide a slow and steady supply of energy without putting an undue stress on your pancreas.

Tacos: For Mexican food lovers, I have some news. Tacos are high in carbohydrates (40 to 50 grams), high in fat (15 to 30 grams), and high in salt content, in the range of 800 to 1200 mg per taco. Moreover, if you consume two tacos, you have enough calories and carbohydrates to keep your body's engine running for the next 24 hours. You are better off eating a chicken or beef fajita with no tortillas and a glass of skim milk or plain water.

Corn products: Corn, being a major carbohydrate ingredient, deserves some comments. One half cup of corn contains roughly 20 grams of carbohydrates and 2 grams of protein. Cornmeal also has a very high GI. Restrict your consumption of cornmeal or corn flakes to no more than 2 ounces per day.

Lean Cuisine: Be aware of Lean Cuisine contents. Most of them emphasize low fat. Do not be misguided by low-fat or fat-free claims. The fat calories may have been replaced by carbohydrate calories. Whether calories come from carbs or fat, they add up! Remember that frozen foods have a much higher salt content than their fresh counterparts. Consider the salt content of frozen foods before you buy them. The sauces and creams used in Lean Cuisine meals are generally made of carbohydrates that add empty calories.

Stay away from packages that contain 60 to 80 grams of carbohydrates. Move to the next aisle, store, or town, where you can select a Lean Cuisine meal with less than 30 grams of carbohydrates. Alternatively, use lunchmeats such as fatless chicken, beef, or turkey to make your own sandwiches. Then add your own vegetables. Become an educated consumer rather than falling prey to such marketing catch phrases as "low-fat" or "fat-free."

I realize that a construction worker digging ditches on the side of the road with his hands, in smoldering 100 degree temperatures for 8 to 10 hours a day, needs many calories. Believe me, he will not be shopping in the Lean Cuisine section. Do not worry about him!

Crackers and cookies: They are a combination of refined carbohydrates and fat. Some of those better-tasting crackers have 150 calories, 14 to 20 grams of carbohydrates, and 6 to 8 grams of fat. Avoid these crackers when you are trying to cultivate a Heart Healthy Lifestyle. In place of crackers, try dry-roasted unsalted soybeans. It will satisfy your appetite, while supplying some nutritious protein, with a small amount of carbohydrates and fat.

Pastries: They look and taste great, and make you feel good. However, are they good for you? These foods are enriched with saturated fats, sugar, and possibly cholesterol. And, of course, they are rich in calories! For example, a croissant has almost 300 calories. The story is the same with most other pastries. Hence, cut your carbohydrate and fat calories by minimizing the pastries in your diet.

Snacks: The basic formula for a snack is some form of carbohydrate cooked in oil. A bag of potato chips contains 30 grams of carbohydrates, 10 to 12 grams of fat, and more than 200 calories. However, a baked version may have very little fat.

Conclusion: Carbohydrates do provide quick energy. Contrary to the conventional wisdom that 50% to 60% of our calories should come from carbohydrates, they are not essential for survival. The human body can manufacture carbohydrates from other sources. Much of the obesity problem in this country is related to overindulgence in carbohydrates and fat-rich foods. As a first step toward a Heart Healthy Lifestyle, I would recommend that you take a serious look at your pantry and carbohydrate inventory. Second, replace most of your higher GI carbohydrate foods with lower GI carbohydrates. Next, reduce your daily carbohydrate consumption to about 50 to 100 grams. Finally, eat most of your carbohydrates in the form of fruits and vegetables.

Notes:

Chapter 04

Proteins
The building blocks of the body

What Are Proteins?

Definition: Proteins are essential for building muscles and cells and replenishing losses through enzyme secretion or breakdown of body tissue. They are also important components of our blood and immune system.

The amino acids are the building blocks of proteins. Each protein may have a chain of hundreds of amino acids. There are two kinds of amino acids, namely essential and non-essential. The body can produce non-essential amino acids from other raw materials. However, the essential amino acids have to come from either plant or animal sources in our diet.

Protein sources: The two major sources of dietary proteins are meat and vegetables. Meat proteins are called complete proteins, since they have all the essential amino acids. Meats also provide vitamins and minerals. Ironically, even though we are eating meat fibers, there is hardly any dietary fiber in meat products. However, be aware that meat contains a large amount of saturated fat, which is harmful to your heart and arteries.

Vegetable sources of proteins such as beans and lentils also contain a certain small amount of fat. In addition, they also contain almost twice the amount of carbohydrates per gram of protein. Unlike the meat protein sources, the beans and lentils, with their skins, provide a good source of fiber. So, a bowl of bean soup contains proteins, carbohydrates, fibers, minerals, and vitamins. The carbohydrates that come from the beans are low glycemic index (GI) carbs, and therefore, they do not raise blood sugar levels as rapidly as white flour, potatoes, or white rice would do.

Protein metabolism: Why can't we take the right type of protein for a given condition? For example, if you want to build muscles, why not take muscle protein that can directly build muscles? When you take in any protein-containing product, the body first breaks the protein down into its smallest components, namely amino acids. The body utilizes these amino acids to make all types of proteins needed for building muscles, making blood cells, repairing tissues, and replacing skin and hair. During periods of starvation, the body breaks down muscle proteins to provide energy for survival. Therefore, crash diets with severely reduced caloric and protein intake can be harmful.

Daily protein requirements: Unlike carbohydrates, you do need a certain amount of protein to maintain normal tissue growth and tissue repair. The American Dietetic Association recommends about 0.8 grams of protein per kilogram (2.2 lbs) of body weight. The total protein intake for an adult weighing 70 kilograms would be approximately 56 grams per day. Construction workers or athletes, who are involved in heavy labor, may require up to 2 grams of protein per kilogram body weight.

Roughly, one ounce of lean meat contains 10 grams of protein. The American Heart Association recommends no more than 8 ounces (0.5 lb) of meat per day. Limit your protein intake to no more 4 ounces (0.25 lb) of meat per meal. Selecting lean cuts of meat and grilling them will further reduce the fat, as the fat will drip down during cooking. Multigrain products are an excellent source of vegetable proteins and a good source of many essential amino acids. Try to get half of your daily protein requirements through vegetable sources such as beans or lentils, which do not contain the same quantity of saturated fats that come with meats.

Then there are the pure or almost pure protein products that predominantly contain protein. Lean chicken breast without skin, lean ground turkey with less than 1% fat, and pure soy protein are some examples.

An average American diet with 2000 calories has 15% of the calories coming from proteins. That translates into 300 calories or roughly 75 grams of protein. But, if you are on a restricted calorie intake as part of your weight control program, you can increase your protein intake to as much as 25% of the total calories without any harmful effect. For example, if you are on 1600 calories, 400 calories can come from proteins. That is equal to 100 grams of protein per day. However, according to the American Diabetes Association, you should restrict your protein intake to 0.8 to 1.0 gram of protein per kilogram body weight. In patients with kidney disease, the protein intake has to be reduced accordingly. Also, people who are on a high protein diet over a prolonged period of time might experience calcium loss and osteoporosis that can lead to bone fractures.

Animal Sources of Proteins

Beef: It is an excellent source of protein. Depending upon the part of the body that it comes from, it may have varying degrees of saturated fat. Four ounces of lean beef contain 25 to 30 grams of protein. The fat content can range anywhere from 6 to 30 grams. Each gram of fat has 9 calories, as opposed to 4 calories coming from proteins. This underscores the importance of keeping the fat content in meat to a minimum.

Even though the American Heart Association recommends drastically reducing red meat in your diet, there is no conclusive evidence that red meat is any more harmful than chicken or fish. However, eating beef or meat products daily is not recommended, as you end up getting excess saturated fats that come with meat products.

Is chicken better than beef? Both chicken and beef provide a good source of protein. Both contain fat, which can vary considerably, especially if the chicken, with its skin and visible yellow fat (saturated fat), is fried. On the other hand, chicken breast has the least amount of fat compared with most other sources of meat products.

Turkey: This is also an excellent source of protein. It is available in many forms with minimal fat content.

Fish: It also provides a good source of protein. Certain types of fish also have health-promoting omega-3 fatty acids. Catfish has more fat compared to other types of fish. Salmon, mackerel, and tuna fish are rich in omega-3s. Omega-3s are polyunsaturated fatty acids, which are known to lower cholesterol. The American Heart Association recommends 2 to 3 servings of fish per week. The best option would be to grill your fish rich in omega-3s for your dinner.

Sausage: A regular sausage is high in saturated fat and calories. Try Healthy Choice sausages that have lower fat content and fewer calories. Sausages made from vegetable products such as soy protein, mushrooms, or vegetables are a very good source of protein with a limited amount of fat. You can find these products in the frozen breakfast section. They come in links or patties.

Ground meat: A regular hamburger patty may have more than 50% of its weight as fat, which contributes to more than 70% of the calories. In addition, it has a high percentage of saturated fats. It may seem reasonable if ground turkey has 7% fat. However, that fat will account for 50% of the total calories. Then you have a choice of ground turkey with 1% fat or ostrich meat that has 3% fat by weight. Another important point to keep in mind is that water accounts for more than 80% of the meat by weight.

Lunchmeats: Lunchmeats are good source of protein with a minimal fat content. They do have a tiny amount of nitrates used as preservatives. Each slice has 1 ounce of meat with 8 to 12 grams of high-quality protein. You can use 2 to 3 slices to provide you with 15 to 20 grams of excellent protein with minimal fat intake. Combine your salads and fruits with your lunchmeat and you have one of the best lightweight, heart healthy lunches that you can carry with you wherever you go. Look for meats that are fat-free, which can further reduce the calorie intake.

Eggs: I will discuss eggs in more detail in the breakfast chapter. Note that egg white is an excellent source of pure protein. You can combine boiled egg whites with other vegetable preparations to increase your protein intake.

Vegetable Sources of Protein

Nuts: They also are a good source of protein. However, they also contain 40% to 50% fat by weight, contributing to 60% or 70% of the total calories. Peanuts have polyunsaturated fatty acids, while macadamia nuts contain a high percentage of calories coming from fats. As a cardiologist, I do not recommend an indiscriminate use of fats. Remember that nuts pack more energy in relationship to their size when compared with other food products.

Thus, moderation is the key when it comes to consumption of nuts. In reality, this is a very challenging task, as most people can't resist emptying a bottle of peanuts once it is opened. I don't know of anyone who can stop at only nine peanuts at a setting. It is more like a bottle of peanuts before the first quarter of the game is finished. If you don't have the willpower, try packing one ounce of nuts in small plastic bags and reward yourself with one packet of nuts from time to time. Macadamia nuts have 50% more fat compared to most other nuts.

On the other hand, dry-roasted soybeans have the least amount of fat compared with most other nuts. My recommendation would be to use dry-roasted soy nuts. You can buy them from health food stores. Keep a packet of soybeans at your workplace or in your car, so you can munch on them when you are hungry and on the run. The soy nuts contain nutritional protein, some carbohydrates, and a limited amount of polyunsaturated fats. Soy nuts are supposed to have estrogen-like compounds that may be concern for women with certain type of breast cancer or in the male population. Since the amount of nuts consumed may be very small, it is unlikely to have noticeable symptoms.

Beans and lentils: There are parts of the world where people primarily depend on the vegetable sources of protein for living. Beans and lentils are the main protein sources in this group. The vegetable proteins have lower fat content compared to the meat products. They also contain fiber, which is not available with meat products. However, most beans and lentils also have carbs as part of their structure. Therefore, it is important to consider the carbs hidden in beans and lentils when you calculate your total carb calories. Take, for example, a can of chickpeas. It has 280 calories, 17.5 grams of protein, 39 grams of carbs, and 10 grams of fiber. Don't forget the oil that you add to season these beans and lentils. Refined beans have more carbohydrate calories than regular beans. They also contain extra salt.

Soy protein: This type of protein has been shown to be beneficial in the prevention and treatment of heart disease, bone disease (osteoporosis), kidney disease and possibly even several types of cancer, including breast cancer. Soy contains more protein when compared to milk, without the saturated fat or cholesterol. Soybeans are the only beans considered to be a complete protein in the vegetable category, as they include all eight essential amino acids. Soy is a low-glycemic index food, which helps in regulating blood sugar and insulin levels. This helps to reduce hunger until your next meal, which is beneficial for weight management. It also lowers LDL (bad) cholesterol and triglycerides. Soy is available in many forms such as beans, milk, sausage, patties, and tofu.

Meat analogs: Many types of meat analogs are available to substitute for ground beef in your hamburgers. These meat analogs are made from soy protein, vegetable sources, rice proteins, and others. You can still continue to enjoy a hamburger from time to time and still maintain a heart healthy lifestyle, if you substitute your regular burger patties with meat analogs or even ground turkey with the least amount of fat.

Harmful effects of proteins: Overindulgence in protein can be harmful. Excess protein intake puts an undue burden on the kidney, with nitrogen overload leading the kidney damage. In addition, we need to be concerned about the excess fat that accompanies protein intake, especially from the animal sources. High protein intake also has been associated with increased calcium elimination in the urine. Increased calcium loss could lead to osteoporosis.

Chapter 05

A Big Fat Story
Plenty of it to digest

What can I say about fat? If I start talking about fat, I am going to enrage half the readers, and if I don't say enough about fat, I will be disappointing the others. Let me bring out some of the factual features of fat, while delicately walking a thin line, to enrich your knowledge about fats and how they interact with your body.

Role of body fat: Body fat serves many useful purposes. It acts as an insulator and a source of energy during periods of prolonged starvation. It is also part of our cell membranes, and acts as a vehicle for transportation of vitamins and enzymes from the gut into the bloodstream.

We will be covering the two components of fats, namely, body fat and dietary fat. In the body, fat is an important element which provides the beautiful and graceful curves that identify you as a person. Dietary fat provides richness, taste, and texture to your foods. When you mix butter or saturated fat with sugar and cholesterol, you have a perfect combination of ingredients for an all-American dessert. Add a few nuts, with lots of fat calories, and we have a mouth-watering recipe than can satisfy any age group. However, the real question is, "Is it heart healthy?" It is anything but heart healthy. Therefore, you need thorough knowledge regarding the true quality and the right quantity of fat that promotes a Heart Healthy Lifestyle.

There are indeed essential fatty acids such as omega-3s and monounsaturated fatty acids, which favorably alter the fat composition of the blood.

Somehow, we have developed a romantic relationship with fat in our diet. The more saturated the fat, the more intense is our relationship with fat. The food industry, having capitalized on this human affinity toward saturated fats, tries to entice consumers into using their brand by enriching their product lines with fats such as lard, butter, coconut or palm oils that are high in saturated fats, which are very harmful to your cardiovascular system. Let's look at the various types of dietary fats that are presently available and how to choose the right fat in your diet.

Dietary fat comes from both animal and plant sources. The animal sources of fat are the visible and invisible fat in the meat. Chicken skin also contains a certain amount of fat.

Reduce the amount of saturated fatty acids. Any fat that is solid at room temperature and is visible to your eyes on your meat products should be removed and discarded. Decrease or minimize the saturated fats in your refrigerator or pantry. You cannot eat what you do not readily have in your refrigerator or your pantry. Increasing your intake of mono- and polyunsaturated fatty acids in proportion to the total fat intake has been shown to reduce the cholesterol level and improve the lipid profile. Keep your fat intake to less than 50 grams per day.

Creams add a great deal of taste, texture, and consistency in addition to acting as lubricants for other food ingredients such as pasta, noodles, etc. Most of these creams are saturated fat emulsions packed with many calories. Whipping cream, rich in saturated fat, is commonly used in Indian cooking to give the rich, tasty gravy texture. Replace your creams rich in saturated fats with low-fat yogurt or non-fat yogurt. You also can use tomato paste to provide the same creamy or gravy-like texture to your food preparations.

Nomenclature of Dietary Fats

Most dietary sources of fat come from milk, dairy products, butter, nuts, beans, and vegetable oils. These fats can be in liquid or solid form. They are also classified on the basis of whether the fats are saturated or unsaturated. Saturation is a process where hydrogen is added to the fatty acids to increase their consistency and shelf life.

Monounsaturated fat: Monounsaturated fatty acids (MUFAs) are probably considered the healthiest type of fat. They do not have the adverse effects of saturated fats, trans fatty acids, or omega-6 polyunsaturated vegetable oils. Oils high in monounsaturated fatty acids are better oils for cooking.

The lower incidence of heart disease in the Mediterranean region is attributed to the high consumption of olive oil and other food products rich in MUFA. MUFA reduces blood cholesterol levels in addition to providing essential fatty acids for healthy skin and development of body cells. Consumption of MUFA has also been associated with a lower incidence of breast and colon cancer. The high vitamin E content of MUFA-rich oils acts as an antioxidant that protects cell damage. Western diets are low in antioxidants. Cold-pressed extra-virgin olive oil, in addition to containing a high percentage of MUFAs, provides a range of phytochemicals (plant-derived chemicals that protect the body) and phenols that boost immunity. MUFAs remain liquid at room temperature, and they can stay fresh for months without getting rancid. However, they become solid when refrigerated.

Oil Source	MUFA	Oil Source	MUFA
Olive oil	73%	Brazil nuts	26%
Rapeseed oil	60%	Cashews	28%
Hazelnuts	50%	Avocado	50%
Almonds	35%	Sesame	20%

Polyunsaturated fatty acids: Polyunsaturated fatty acids (PUFAs) have more than one unsaturated bond, where hydrogen atoms can be added to make them saturated fatty acids (SFAs). Most PUFAs come from vegetable sources. They remain liquid at room temperature and in the refrigerator. The PUFAs can easily combine with oxygen in the air and turn rancid. Hence, it is very important to keep your PUFAs in dark, closed containers when not used. If you use PUFAs for frying, make sure that you use the least amount of oil needed and discard the oil after one use. Repeated heating of PUFAs turns them into trans fatty acids that increase the risk of heart disease. The PUFAs have been shown to lower blood cholesterol levels.

PUFAs also improve insulin sensitivity. Excess saturated fat intake increases insulin resistance, which means more insulin will be needed to control a given level of blood sugar. A diet rich in PUFAs in place of SFAs have been shown to lower blood pressure. Therefore, regular fish (a rich source of PUFA) consumption could lead to lower blood pressure.

Margarine is produced by hydrogenating oils containing PUFAs, which increases both the SFA and trans fatty acid content. Recently, U.S. Food and Drug Administration (FDA) regulations require manufacturers to list the trans fatty acid content in their food preparations. Today, most snacks sold in the grocery stores have less than 0.5 grams of trans fatty acids.

Saturated fatty acids: SFAs have all the hydrogen and the carbon atoms they can hold. Usually, saturated fats are solid at room temperature. Unlike the PUFAs, the SFAs do not readily combine with the oxygen in the air, thus making them more stable. The SFAs raise the total and LDL cholesterol levels. Most of the SFAs come from animal sources. The visible fat in and around the meat contains SFAs. Choose fats and oils that contain <2 grams of saturated fat per tablespoon. The dietaary sources of saturated fats to watch are: coconut oil, butter, cheese, creams, and dairy products.

Thrombosis or blood clotting contribute to arterial blockage. High fat intake has been associated with increased platelet stickiness that can lead to clot formation.

Hydrogenated fats: Most vegetable oils are liquid at room temperature. To increase their shelf-life and make them more palatable, hydrogen atoms are added to the liquid oils (a process called hydrogenation). This process of hydrogenation turns the PUFAs into fatty acids with a higher proportion of SFAs. The greater the degree of hydrogenation, the more saturated the fat becomes. Margarine is an example of a fat containing partially hydrogenated fats derived from PUFAs. The hydrogenated fats raise cholesterol levels more than their PUFA precursors.

Trans fatty acids: Hydrogenation of PUFAs, like heating, leads to the formation of trans fatty acids (TFAs). TFAs raise the total and LDL (bad) cholesterol levels and decrease the HDL cholesterol levels. They are attractive to restaurant chiefs because they provide taste, richness, and texture to foods. TFAs are used in the preparation of many cookies, crackers, and bakery items. Pay attention to the labels on ready-made pastries, cookies, snacks, or crackers, looking for the TFA content. French fries, donuts, and other commercial fried foods are major sources of TFAs in your diet.

TFAs result from an anaerobic bacterial fermentation in ruminant animals and thereby enter the main food chain. We eat them as meat and dairy products. It is estimated that our daily intake of TFAs ranges from 2.6 to 12.8 grams. The TFAs have also been shown to increase the levels of lipoprotein(a), which has a direct relationship to the coronary artery disease incidence. The higher the level of lipoprotein(a), the greater the incidence of coronary artery disease. The effect of TFAs on triglyceride levels is highly variable.

A Common-Sense Approach

This approach would dictate the use of MUFAs and PUFAs in place of TFAs or SFAs whenever possible. Additionally, substituting softer margarines for harder margarines seems justified.

It is important to realize that strict dietary fat reduction can lower your total cholesterol level by as much as 20 to 25 mg%. However, if your total cholesterol level is in the range of 275 mg% or more, do not expect your diet modification alone to reduce your total cholesterol to the desired level. You have to engage in a vigorous exercise program in addition to possibly taking some cholesterol lowering medicines. Refer to the chapter on lowering your cholesterol level naturally.

Even with many diet programs, you may not be able to drastically reduce your total fat intake over extended periods. However, the knowledge provided here can make you an educated consumer, so you can not only reduce your total fat intake, but also at the same time alter the composition of your fat intake in a favorable manner, thus reducing your risk of heart disease in the long run.

When you replace your SFAs and TFAs with carbohydrate-based products, they may decrease the total cholesterol at the expense of increasing your triglyceride levels. Hence, the key is to reduce fat intake, carbs, and overall total calories. You should place more emphasis on consumption of MUFAs, PUFAs, and omega-3s than on a total elimination of SFAs or TFAs from your diet.

Presently, 12% to 15% of our daily calories come from saturated fats. If you are on a 3000-calorie diet, it amounts to 450 calories coming from saturated fats or 50 grams of saturated fat per day. The American Heart Association recommends no more than 10% of your total calories coming from saturated fats. In patients with severe cholesterol problems, even a reduction of total intake of all types of fats to about 15% may be necessary to achieve the optimal total and LDL cholesterol levels.

Consumption of soybean oil and semi-liquid margarine can lower total cholesterol and LDL levels to a greater degree than the consumption of solid margarine, shortening, or butter.

Ketones: Most people assume that ketones are bad. Ketones are neither bad nor good as long as they are self-contained. Severe ketosis, noted during extreme degrees of starvation, can be harmful. On the other hand, you need to understand the basic biochemical mechanism by which our body mobilizes the fat from its large fat deposits. Ketones are the byproducts of fat breakdown. Hence, ketones are produced whether you are on a low carb, low protein, low-fat, or high-fat diet, as long as your body has to break down fat for calories and energy. The body has better control over how much body fat it has to mobilize at any given time to provide energy. When we eat fatty foods, we may not have such control. When you overload your body with an enormous amount of fat from the diet (following a juicy steak dinner at a lavish reception), ketone bodies will be produced during the breakdown of larger fat particles into smaller, more digestible fatty acids or triglycerides.

When you are on a restricted carbohydrate diet with unlimited fat intake, you are increasing the amount of fat available from both inside and outside the body for energy needs. This excess fat breakdown leads to more ketone production. In order to have an orderly fat breakdown, the key is to reduce your total calorie intake, including the amount of fat in your diet. That forces your body to mobilize the internal fat on a needed basis for energy, thus minimizing severe ketosis while at the same time promoting the mobilization of body fat. That is our goal in losing weight to begin with.

Daily fat intake: The American Heart Association recommends that 30% of your daily calories come from fat. It also recommends no more than 10% of total calories to come from saturated fats. According to the table below, you will notice that the total fat calories vary depending on the total calories. So, you may want to pay special attention to the total calories and grams of fat.

Keeping Your Fat Intake to 30% of Total Calories

Total Diet Calories	Total Fat	Fat calories	Fat, grams
3000	30%	1000	111
2400	30%	800	89
1800	30%	540	50
1200	30%	360	40

If you take a different approach and reduce your fat intake to 15%, 10%, or even 7% of your total calories, you will notice the total grams that you have to live by.

Fat Restricted Diets

Total Calories	Total Fat	Fat, calories	Fat, grams
2000	30%	600	67
2000	15%	300	33
2000	10%	200	22
2000	7%	140	15

As the total fat intake gets lower and lower, the chances of staying on that diet over an extended period become very slim. That is one of the reasons why I think it is better to reduce the total calorie intake than trying to severely restrict your fat percentage.

If you are trying to lose weight or trying to aggressively lower your cholesterol, reducing your calorie intake will lower your fat intake much more effectively. Therefore, I would suggest keeping your total fat intake to less than 50 grams per day or 450 calories. Adjust your carbs to meet the extra caloric requirements.

Dietary Fat Classification

Dietary Fat	Sources
MUFA	Olive, canola and peanut oils, avocados
PUFA	Safflower, sesame, soy, corn and sunflower-seed oils, nuts and seeds
SFA	Whole milk, cream, ice cream, whole-milk cheeses, butter, lard and meats. Palm, palm kernel and coconut oils
TFA	Cookies, crackers, cakes, French fries, fried onion rings, donuts
Cholesterol	Meats, egg yolks, dairy products, organ meats (heart, etc.), shrimp and poultry

Low-Fat and Low-Carbohydrate Myths

One diet expert advocates unlimited fat intake while another one recommends you to lower your fat intake to <10% of your daily calories. The real question is—can you live on either of these diets all your life? Most Americans consume 30% to 40% of their calories as fat. I don't believe it is practical to live on a rigid low-fat diet, with <10% of your calories coming from fat. With the modern cholesterol lowering drugs that can reduce your cholesterol by as much as 50%, there is no need to live on a fat-starvation diet. I did not mean to advocate, "Enjoy your steak and take your pills." I just wanted to emphasize the unrealistic expectations of a diet that is supposed to last you a lifetime.

I have talked to many people who were on unlimited fat diets in the past. Their most resounding comments were "Finally, I got sick of that bacon, sausage, and all that grease." Of course, when you talk to people who did not like what they were doing, they are going to have negative and sometimes antagonistic feelings toward the program that did not help them to achieve their goal (sustained weight loss). There is some truth to both sides of the story.

Most cardiologists and I feel indiscriminate dietary fat intake can be harmful. Numerous studies have shown a direct relationship between increased saturated fat intake and increased heart disease risk. In fact, people who go on a low-fat diet (for example, decreasing their fat intake from 40% of calories to 30% of calories) have decreased their total cholesterol, their LDL cholesterol, and their cholesterol ratio favorably.

You can test this hypothesis yourself by testing your lipid levels before and after you have been on a low-calorie, low-fat diet. If the numbers change favorably, which I have noticed in most of my patients, then you know that your diet is working. There are some instances where I have not seen any improvement, in people who just cannot stick to their new diet and lifestyle. That is reality, which both the patient and I have to resolve. If I unreasonably force that person to stick to my dogmatic view, he will seek the path of least resistance—find a new doctor. That defeats the very point I am trying to convey—practicality.

Fat substitutes: Fat substitutes are ingredients that mimic one or more of the roles of fat in a food. They are classified into three categories based on their nutrient source. Carbohydrate-based fat substitutes use plant polysaccharides in place of fat. Proteins and microparticulated proteins are used as fat replacers. Fat-based fat replacers act as barriers to block fat absorption.

How are fat substitutes used? Fat substitutes have been developed to decrease the quantity of fat in foods and help people lower their fat intake. Some fat replacers are used as fat substitutes or fat analogs and replace fat in a food. Others are used as fat mimetics to partially replace fat and give the sensory qualities of fat (taste and feel in the mouth).

Some evidence suggests that people who include fat-modified products in their diet may have a reduced fat and calorie intake and improved nutrient profile compared with people who don't use any fat-modified products.

Are fat substitutes safe and helpful? Fat-modified products have been introduced into the food supply recently and only affect a few foods so far. Although fat substitutes on the market are considered safe by the FDA, their long-term benefits and safety are not known. Still, within the context of a healthy diet that meets dietary recommendations, fat substitutes used appropriately can provide flexibility with diet planning.

When selecting a fat substitute, consider its effect on your blood lipids, as well its calories and availability. Taste should be an important consideration, as most of us cannot live on an artificial and tasteless diet for very long. Even the most stringent fat restriction is not going to bring your cholesterol down from, say, 300 to 200 mg%. The most you can expect is to reduce your cholesterol by 20 mg% to 30 mg%. Carbohydrate-based products add more calories to your diet. Protein-based products may not stimulate your insulin production, but increase the nitrogen in your diet. Select low-calorie dressings in place of regular salad dressings (a low-calorie dressing may have 20 calories in comparison to a regular dressing that may have 15 to 20 grams of fat and 150 to 200 calories).

Reheating cooking oil more than once will lead to the formation of TFAs that act as saturated fats.

Once, I removed more than 100 grams of oil from chicken gravy. It was more than the oil that was initially used to season the onions and the chicken.

When you cook meat, it releases the hidden fat that floats at the top like a clear liquid. You can use a simple siphon to remove all the floating oil from your food preparations. These simple and common-sense steps will enable you to minimize the oil in your diet while at the same time enabling you to enjoy the foods that you love to relish.

Choices for Fats

Use olive oil for salad dressing, cooking, marinating meat, and baking. Soy oil, safflower oil and canola are also good alternatives.

Select Benecol or Take Control, which have plant sterol and stanols, in place of regular margarine.

Use low-fat milk in place of regular milk.

Minimize the use of butter and coconut oil, as they contain a high percentage of SFAs.

Limit the consumption of nuts to one ounce, which will give you 12 to 14 grams of PUFA.

Trim all visible fat from meat before you cook it.

Grill your meat so that most of the oil will drip off it, into the grill.

Remove any visible oil or fat from your cooked foods before serving.

Select lean ground meat that has less than 3 to 7% fat.

Try adding a tablespoon of flaxseed to your salad or breakfast cereal. It is rich in omega-3s that are good for our body, as they reduce cholesterol levels. Another option is to use fish oil capsules that are rich in omega-3s.

Consider using oils such as olestra, which recently have been used for snacks with the hope that their large fatty acids would not be absorbed by the intestines. Some people may complain of bloating and diarrhea.

Use reduced-fat or no-fat salad dressings with salads, for dips or as a marinade.

Remember to count the "hidden fat" in bakery and snack foods as well as the fats used in cooking and on vegetables and breads.

Notes:

Chapter 06

Desi Foods, Calorie Counts & Vegetarian Myths
Not all diets are created equal

Desi Foods & Calorie Counts

Since I am from India, I see many people from my subcontinent, including Pakistan, Sri Lanka, Bangladesh, Nepal, and a few other countries. We have very similar food habits, risk factors, and clusters of diseases indigenous to our region. Hence, I have devoted this chapter to Desi (a term that refers to people from the above countries) food styles. Most of the information applies to people of other ethnic groups and the references are based on raw food products and their compositions.

If you are trying to get an approximate calorie count and composition of Desi foods for a weight loss, diabetic, high blood pressure, or low-cholesterol diet for heart risk reduction, here is a rough guide to some cooked and many raw ingredients used in Desi cooking.

You don't have to be a diet expert or a nutritionist to know when you are eating the wrong kinds of Desi foods. Take a look at some choices:

When there is more oil than a plate can hold, you are eating the wrong food. An example? Curry.

When the food tastes sweeter than sugar and richer than butter, then you are eating the wrong food—desserts.

When you have eaten two or three plates of rice, and you are still hungry, you need help.

When you have to loosen your belt by two inches, then you have eaten too much of the wrong foods (all of the above).

Now, knowing what we are doing is wrong, let us concentrate on learning a leaner and trimmer dietary habit for a heart healthy lifestyle. You don't have to be a rocket scientist to craft out a simple heart healthy diet. However, you need to understand the "Desi Diet 101" principles and guidelines.

First, let's concentrate on counting the approximate calorie counts from the raw foods used in Desi cooking. Next, we'll look at some commonly prepared foods in terms of calorie, protein, fat, and carbohydrate contents.

Let's say you or a member of your family is on a special diet for diabetes or heart disease. Then you need to understand that all food we eat has energy stored in it as calories. Energy comes from three major ingredients in our foods: carbohydrates, proteins, and fats. The source of these ingredients does not matter (vegetarian or non-vegetarian) as far as the calories are concerned.

Before we can calculate the calorie counts of our commonly used foods, we need to have an understanding of simple measurements of our foods.

One teaspoon holds	5 grams
One tablespoon is equal to	15 ml
One ounce is equal to	30 grams
One cup holds	240 ml

Each gram of carbohydrates and proteins has 4 calories while each gram of fat has 9 calories. Let's look at some real-life examples:

One cup of uncooked rice has 240 grams of carbohydrates and 960 calories (240 grams x 4 calories per gram). The same calculation applies for flour used for all types of breads, naans, parathas, and chapatis. When we talk about carbohydrates, we need to keep in mind the glycemic index, which tells us which foods raise your blood sugar level quickly. Foods with a high glycemic index may have an adverse effect on your insulin demand, especially in diabetic patients.

Half a cup of butter (120 ml) has 1080 calories (120 x 9). The same principle applies to all types of vegetable oils. Animal fat contains more saturated fats, which are bad. Refer to the chapter on, "A Big Fat story."

Raw foods such as chicken or meat have lots of water, and hence, the calorie count does not match with their weight. A lean skinless boneless 4.7 ounce portion of chicken breast has 160 calories, 28 grams of protein, and 5 grams of fat. Four ounces of lean lamb leg has 205 calories, 31 grams of protein, and 8 grams of fat. Similar approximations can be made to other meats, provided they are skinless, boneless, and fat-trimmed.

Among the vegetable sources, half a cup of chickpeas contains 120 calories, 5 grams of protein, 20 grams of carbohydrates, 2.5 grams of fat, and 5 grams of fiber.

One large potato (5.6 oz.) contains 100 calories, 4 grams of protein, and 26 grams of carbohydrates.

One ounce of peanuts contains 170 calories, 7 grams of protein, 6 grams of carbohydrates, and 14 grams of fat. Other nuts have similar compositions.

One cup of regular milk (8 oz.) contains 160 calories, 9 grams of protein, 12 grams of carbohydrates, and 8 grams of fat. If you use skim milk, you can eliminate the 8 grams of fat and reduce the calorie count by 50%, to 80 calories.

Let's calculate the composition of a chicken curry and rice dinner. Let's begin with raw ingredients and their approximate calories:

One cup of rice with 240 grams of carbohydrates contains approximately 960 calories.

You choose chicken leg quarters for curry since the chicken breast may be too dry. One pound of skinless chicken leg quarters (16 ounces) contains approximately 900 calories, 80 grams of protein, and 64 grams of fat. Let us assume you use 120 ml of vegetable oil for cooking, adding another 1080 calories. One big onion provides 30 calories from carbohydrates. Six ounces of tomatoes add 40 calories from 8 grams of carbohydrates.

This dinner composition includes 3130 calories (960+900+ 1080+70). The total composition includes 256 grams of carbohydrates, 80 grams of protein, and 184 grams of fat.

Let's analyze this diet from a nutritional point of view. If we divide this diet into 4 servings, each serving will have 64 grams of carbohydrates, 20 grams of protein, a whopping 50 grams of fat, and 783 calories.

This is a very modest diet portion by any Desi standard. How can we make this heart healthy? The major culprit here seems to be the fats that we use in our Desi cooking. We have no concept of how calories add up when we use oil indiscriminately in our cooking. If we were to reduce the oil used by 60 ml, we would reduce the total calories to 648, and the total fat intake to 35 grams per serving.

Our daily intake of carbohydrates should be less than 200 grams, proteins 50 to 70 grams and fats less than 50 grams.

Consider grilling your meat instead of making a gravy. The gravy is basically a fat emulsion containing vegetables, vegetable oil, or worst yet, whipping cream that has 50% saturated fats.

There is no single source of comprehensive calorie count on all cooked Indian foods, since there is such a wide variation in the cooking methods and the quality of oil used in the preparation of foods with similar names such as chicken curry, lamb korma, or biryani. However, using the tables in this article, you can get an approximate calorie count and the amount of fat in each raw ingredient.

The two major ingredients that add excess calories are carbohydrates and fats. If you can cut down on your carbohydrates and fat in your daily cooking based on these tables, you can indeed prepare tasty Desi delights to entice your taste buds.

Dairy products: They are an excellent balanced food consisting of carbohydrates, proteins, and fats.

Dairy Products, Eggs, and Cheese				
8 oz. Serving	Cal	C, g	P, g	F, g
Milk, whole	150	12	8	8
Milk, 2%	130	13	8	5
Skim milk	80	12	9	0
Milk chocolate	240	33	8	9

Half & Half, 1 Tbsp	40	1	1	3
Whipping cream, 1 cup	699	7	5	74
Sour cream, 1 cup	493	10	7	48
Yogurt, fat-free	130	19	12	0
Eggs	80	1	7	4.5
Whole-wheat bread	50	10	4	1
Swiss cheese	70	0	5	5
Cal = calories, C = carbs, P = proteins, F = fats, g = grams				

Consider skim milk in your preparations if you want to reduce your fat intake. The glycemic index of skim milk is much less than that of rice or potatoes.

Creams used in gravy are very high in fats. Consider tomatoes and fat-free yogurt for your gravy. Better yet, reduce the amount of gravy that you cook. Buttermilk is an excellent source of protein. Use diluted buttermilk as your soft drink during hot summer months.

Carbohydrates: They are the main source of calories in the Desi diet. They are also the worst enemy of the Desi diet, as we have an addiction when it comes to carbohydrates in terms of rice, naan, or parathas.

While we are on the subject of carbohydrates, we need to consider the glycemic index (GI) of foods. The GI tells us how quickly a given carbohydrate will raise your blood sugar compared to that when you consume pure glucose. The lower the GI, the slower that your blood sugar rises and the less fluctuation in your insulin levels. Select foods that have a GI of less than 50 wherever you can. For example, the GI of parboiled rice is 72 compared to 52 for brown rice, or 53 for Basmati rice. Similarly, the GI of baked potato is 85. Potatoes just add empty calories and raise your blood sugar quickly.

Carbohydrate Rich Foods				
100 g Serving	Cal	C, g	P, g	F, g
Wheat flour	341	70	12	1.7
Rice	346	80	6.4	0.4
Bengal gram	372	60	20	5.6

Black gram	347	60	24	1.4
Peas	315	57	20	1.1
Potatoes	97	23	1.6	1
Bananas	116	27	1.2	1
Dates	317	76	2.5	1
Apples	90	22	-	-
Pears	100	25	1	-
Grapefruit	60	16	1	-
Onions, 3 oz	30	7	1	-
Naan	336	50	9	13
Cal = calories, C = carbs, P = proteins, F = fats, g = grams				

Protein-rich choices: There are plenty of good choices available from both vegetarian and non-vegetarian sources. You need at least 50 to 70 grams of protein per day.

Protein Rich Foods				
100 g Serving	Cal	C,g	P, g	F, g
Soybeans	432	21	43	20
Cashews	596	22	21	47
Almonds	655	10	21	59
Cheese	348	6.3	24	25
Prawns	273	2.9	21	20
Shrimp	349	-	68	9
Chicken breast	140	0	25	4
Chicken legs	160	0	19	10
Catfish, 4 oz.	153	0	18	9
Beef, ground lean, 4 oz	290	0	29	19
Tofu, 4 oz	60	2	6	3
Chickpeas, dry ¼ cup	170	29	10	2
Peas	120	20	7	1
Cottage cheese, ½ cup	120	5	13	5
Turkey, lean	193	-	13	6

There are plenty of vegetable sources of proteins. You have

to develop a taste for those foods. Milk products, artificial creams, soybeans, chickpeas, and various types of daal provide good protein.

Fat-rich foods: Fat-rich foods are all around. If you smell good food and it tastes good, you bet it has a lot of fat and sugar. Use olive oil, which has a higher percentage of monounsaturated fatty acids. Avoid whipping cream, plain yogurt, shortening, and lard.

Fat Rich Foods				
1 Tbsp Serving	Cal	C, g	P, g	F, g
Butter	110	-	-	12
Flaxseeds	140	11	5	10
Cashews	596	22	21	47
Almonds	655	10	21	59
Cheese	348	6.3	24	25
Cal = calories, C = carbs, P = proteins, F = fats, g = grams				

Consider Benecol or Total Control margarine for your spreads, as they contain plant sterols and stanols that can reduce total cholesterol. Select skinless and boneless chicken. Trim all visible fat. Use light olive oil to season your vegetables. After preparing gravy, remove all the floating oil.

Restaurant tips: Most Desi restaurants use vegetable oil or whipping cream to provide rich and tasty gravy that is loaded with fat calories. Consider ordering grilled meat such as tandoori, tikka, or lamb chops, instead of chicken butter masala or lamb curry. Use vegetable korma sparingly, as it may have too much fat. Instead, consider mixed seasoned vegetables.

Is a Vegetarian Diet Safe?

Most people believe that a vegetarian diet is good for their heart. What is good for your palate is not necessarily good for your heart. The vegetarian diet is neither good nor bad, depending upon its composition. However, if take a close look at the composition of a typical vegetarian diet, you will notice that it is loaded with excessive amounts of carbohydrates:

Breakfast carbohydrates: breads, dosa, idli, cereals, rice, chapati, naan, potatoes, milk, and fruits.

Lunch carbohydrates: Rice, wheat, chapati, flour, potatoes, peas, naan, milk, and fruits.

Dinner carbohydrates: Naan, chapati, rice, beans, potatoes, sweets, bananas, milk, and fruits.

How Much Carbohydrate Do We Need? With the exception of eggs, meat, and pure butter, just about everything you touch is loaded with carbohydrates. As a result, the Desi vegetarian diet may have 80% of its calories coming from carbohydrates, whereas carbohydrates in most American diets account for 50% to 55% of the total calories. When you consume such an enormous amount of carbohydrates, you are likely to have glucose intolerance and elevated triglycerides, or be overweight.

As mentioned in the chapter on carbohydrates, your body needs about 200 grams of carbohydrates per day. It is interesting to note that your body stores about 400 grams of carbohydrates in the form of glycogen in the liver and muscles to supply the immediate energy needs. For long-term energy needs, your body depends on fatty acids. When you stuff your system with 300 to 600 grams of sugar per day, the body has no choice but to store only a part of it as glycogen, while the rest of it is going to be converted into fatty acids or triglycerides. The triglycerides are now considered an independent risk factor for heart disease. The triglycerides are associated with higher LDL (the bad) cholesterol levels. Now you can see the link between a vegetarian high-carbohydrate diet, triglycerides, elevated LDL levels, and heart disease.

What is the solution? Even though most American diets recommend 1800 to 2400 calories per day, we do not burn that number of calories. Whatever calories we do not burn will turn into fat and LDL cholesterol. The first step in modifying your diet is to reduce the amount of carbohydrates to less than 200 grams per day or perhaps to less than 100 grams per day. The total reduction in calories has multiple benefits, such as reduced sugar levels, lower triglyceride levels, reduced LDL level, weight control, and better diabetes control. You can have a healthy lifestyle by consuming as few as 1200 to 1500 calories per day. There are two main types of carbohydrates based on their glycemic index (GI). The GI refers the rapidity at which your carbohydrate turns into pure glucose in the body. When you consume pure glucose, it is readily available for energy in the body. Hence, it is considered to have a GI of 100. On the other hand, certain fat and meat products have a very low GI. You should select foods that have less than a 50% GI. Please visit www.sugarlandheartcenter.com and look for a chart that has a list of foods along with their (GI) numbers. The lower the GI, the slower the release of sugar. This serves to maintain a steady glucose level without overloading the system and increasing the insulin demand.

What about fats? Fat contains triglycerides, which are the building blocks of fatty tissue in the body. Unlike carbohydrates, which are stored in a finite amount in the body (400 mg in the form of glycogen), there is no limit as to the amount of fat that your body can accumulate. Like a friend of mine said, when it comes to fats, "a second on your lips, and the rest of the time on your hips." That is a very high price to pay, especially when you are having a love affair with sweets and fried foods. The key here is to reduce your fat intake drastically.

According to the American Heart Association, your total fat intake should be less than 30% of your total calories. If you are on a 1500 calorie diet, that amounts to 500 calories, which translates into roughly 55 grams of fat per day. There are different types of fats. Saturated fats are generally solid at room temperature and can lead to high levels of cholesterol. There are poly- and monounsaturated fats that are less harmful. Avoid animal fat, butter, and coconut, which are high in saturated fats. Select olive oil for cooking and minimize fried foods. You can also choose plant sterol and stanol spreads, such as Total Control or Benecol, which reduce your cholesterol levels. Keep your saturated fat intake to less than 10% of the total calories. That means less than 150 calories can come from saturated fats, which amount to 16 to 17 grams of saturated fat, or equal to a tablespoon of saturated fat. It would be very difficult to count such a small quantity of fat, and the simplest solution is to minimize the intake of saturated fats. Remember that the so-called low-fat products may be loaded with carbohydrates to provide the consistency. Read the labels!

Where can I get more proteins? Unlike carbohydrates and fats, which our body has the ability to manufacture, most of our protein has to come from dietary sources. There are 8 essential amino acids, the building blocks of proteins, which have to be provided from dietary sources. The biggest concern that most vegetarians have is how they can increase their protein intake while keeping their carbohydrate intake low. There are plenty of vegetable sources that contain protein. However, you need to understand that most vegetable sources of proteins such as peas and daal also have carbohydrates which need to be taken into consideration while cooking.

Take, for example, a serving of chickpeas. When you read the nutritional label, you will notice that it has 6 grams of protein, but also has 12 grams of carbohydrates. The rule of thumb is that there are twice as many grams of carbohydrates as there are proteins. Nonetheless, there are excellent sources of protein such as eggs without the yolk, cottage cheese, tofu, peas, beans, daals, skim milk, avocado, soybeans, and nuts. One more important point to remember is that most of these products also contain fat. Over 60% of the calories in nuts (peanuts and cashews) come from polyunsaturated fats. Each gram of protein contains 4 calories. The average daily intake of protein should be less than 2 grams per kilogram of body weight, which amounts to less than 150 grams per day.

Do I need to hire a dietitian? You do not need to be an expert dietitian to craft out a heart healthy diet. If you know how to precisely measure the ingredients for a cheesecake or determine the quantity of salt and spices for your favorite biryani, you can calculate the amount of carbs, fat, and protein by simply reading the labels and translating to the amount of carbohydrates, fat, and protein you consume per day. Multiply the carbohydrate or protein grams by 3.5 to get the calories from each group. Multiple the fat grams by 9 to get the calories from your fats. Use that as the starting point, and then systematically reduce the quantity of carbohydrates or fats until you reach a desired calorie count and the right combination of carbohydrates, fat, and proteins (roughly 100 to 200 grams of carbohydrates, 50 grams of fat, and less than 150 grams of protein per day).

If you are preparing for the entire family, measure the amount of dry food such as rice to get the total calories and then divide it by the number of people to arrive at each person's consumption. For example, a cup of dry rice has 240 grams of carbohydrates. That translates into 960 calories (240 x 4). A cup of dry rice turns into 6 cups of cooked rice. If four people eat that rice, each person will get approximately 210 calories from carbohydrates. Similarly, pour the amount of cooking oil you use per day into a measuring cup. Multiply the volume in ml by 9 to get the calories from fat. If you have 50 ml of oil, it accounts for 450 calories (50 x 9)! To that, add all the fat that comes from the nuts, daals, peas, etc. Now you have daily total fat and fat calorie intake.

You give a man a fish, he will eat for a day. You teach a man how to fish, he will eat for the rest of his life. With this short introduction, I have given you tips on how to fish out your heart healthy diet with some simple useful hooks.

Notes:

Chapter 07

Vegetables, Fresh Fruits & Fiber

Vegetables & Fresh Fruits

The other day, a nurse friend of mine, Sandy, grabbed me and asked, "Are you still working on your Heart Healthy Lifestyle book?"

"Why do you ask?" I said.

"Today I heard something about free oxygen radicals causing skin damage." She looked worried.

"I didn't know that you were worried about your skin. I thought that you wanted to lose weight."

"Well, I want to."

"What do you mean by 'Well, I want to'?" I asked.

"If you finish writing your book, maybe I can take a second look at your diet program," she said.

"What do you want to know?" I pressed.

"What are oxygen free radicals?" she quizzed.

"I call them rascals, because they account for most of the skin, organ, and blood vessel damage. The blood vessel damage initiates the hardening (artherosclerosis) process in the arteries that eventually leads to their total blockage, resulting in a heart attack, stroke, or kidney failure. The skin damage leads to wrinkles, loss of texture, and aging." I paused.

"How do I counteract the effects of oxygen free radicals?"

"Free radicals are constantly produced in our body cells during routine metabolic processes of converting food into energy. The free radicals such as superoxide, peroxyl radicals, hydroxyl radicals, and peroxynitrite are very destructive in nature. They cause skin damage, arterial wall damage, and organ damage. The damaging effects of free radicals can be partially neutralized or prevented by regularly supplying antioxidants in our diet."

"How do antioxidants work?"

"Antioxidants attach themselves to the free oxygen radicals and convert them into harmless objects."

"Can you name some antioxidants?" she questioned.

"Vitamin A, C, and E, zinc, magnesium, and selenium have antioxidant properties. Flavonoids also have strong antioxidant properties."

"How do I get these antioxidants?"

"Do you want the easy route or the more practical route?"

"Give me the easy route first. If I don't like it, I don't have to waste my time on the more complicated one!" she said.

"Maybe I should not even have asked the question to begin with. Most drugs stores carry antioxidant formulas. Generally speaking, you can take 2 to 4 capsules per day. But a better way to get your antioxidants is through careful selection of fresh fruits and dark leafy vegetables."

"How do fruits and vegetables come into this picture?"

"That is a good question. Most vitamins and minerals come from plant sources. Fresh fruits and vegetables naturally are excellent sources of antioxidants, minerals, and phytochemicals. Phytochemicals counteract the effect of harmful chemicals. In addition, fresh fruits and vegetables contain fiber, enzymes, and flavonoids."

"Nik, what are flavonoids?" Sandy inquired.

"Flavonoids are a group of chemicals found in some fruits that neutralize the effect of free radicals containing peroxide and superoxide. Flavonoids are also found in darkly pigmented vegetables."

"Can you give me some examples of foods containing flavonoids?"

"Tomatoes, green leafy vegetables, cantaloupes, strawberries, blueberries, raspberries, grapeseeds, and red, yellow or blue bell pepper — just to name a few."

"But, Nik, don't fruits contain sugar?"

"That is an excellent point, and you're right! Most fruits do contain carbohydrates. That is one of the reasons why I recommend my patients to replace part of their breads, rice, and pasta servings with fresh fruits and vegetables."

"Oh! Does that mean no more bread, rice, or pasta?"

"The less you eat of these items, the better it is for your skin, organs, and blood vessels."

"All right, Doc. Now, let me ask you something else. Why do you recommend fresh fruits over fruit juices?"

"Look at their composition. Fruit juices are basically liquid extracts of fruits. When you squeeze a fresh orange or a tangerine, you get orange or tangerine juice. But what you are leaving in the pulp is more important than what is filling the cup! The pulp contains minerals, enzymes, and fiber, among other things. Keep in mind that fruit juices sold in the supermarkets may have added preservatives to increase their shelf life and sugar to enhance their taste. So, let me ask you a question. Would you rather drink just the carbohydrate content of a fruit or have the whole fresh fruit with its complete advantages?"

"That makes sense. Are you saying, go for the fresh fruits whenever there is a choice?"

"Actually, if you do not have a choice, settle for a glass of skim milk instead of bottled fruit juice," I emphasized.

"But I don't like skim milk," Sandy whined. "Why can't I just have the orange juice?"

"Well, let me explain my logic behind this. A glass of fruit juice contains mostly carbohydrates, some of which are pure sugar. On the other hand, 8 ounces of skim milk contain 8 to 9 grams of proteins, 11 grams of carbs, calcium, and zero grams of fat."

"Did you just say there are 11 grams of carbs? What makes these carbs any better than the carbs in fruit juice?" she quizzed.

"Smart question! Fruits contain fructose that has a glycemic index (GI) of 50. No doubt, fruit juice has carbohydrate with a lesser GI than rice or potatoes. However, fruits do not have the protein contained in skim milk. In addition, fruit juices have 25 to 30 grams of carbohydrates while skim milk has only 11 grams of carbohydrates."

"Well, okay, I guess I can see why I should stick to the skim milk."

"Wait a minute! Did you finally think for once that I was right?" I interjected.

"Not exactly, so don't get your hopes up! How do vegetables help us fight against aging and heart disease?"

"Vegetables contain soluble fiber, which lowers blood cholesterol levels. They also add bulk and fill you up more than bread or rice. Best of all, they have less calories compared with carbohydrates or proteins. As I mentioned before, fresh fruits and vegetables have antioxidants that prevent arterial damage and plaque buildup."

"So, what kind of vegetables do you recommend?"

"Select dark green leafy vegetables such as romaine lettuce as part of your daily lunch and dinner meals. The darker the color, the more antioxidants they contain. Add a teaspoon of olive oil, which is known to lower cholesterol, to your salad. Sprinkle a little salt and pepper on it, and squeeze half a lemon on top of that. Now you have the best salad in town."

"That's it?"

"Oh! Did I mention slices of red and yellow bell peppers?"

"But, Nik, you must be out of your mind! Most of us do not have time to prepare salads for lunch and dinner."

"You bring up an excellent point. That is why God created weekends. Select dark green leafy vegetables, colorful bell peppers, and all kinds of berries on your weekend shopping trips to the supermarket. Spend a few minutes on Sunday afternoons, after returning from your lunch, to chop up the leafy vegetables, bell peppers, and mix those ingredients with the berries. Divide the salad into daily portion servings and fill Ziploc bags with the salad. When you come home from work each day, take out one packet of this salad mixture from the fridge, add to it salt and pepper, a teaspoon of olive oil, and lemon juice. How long is this going to take you to prepare — maybe one minute? Two minutes? Or three minutes?"

"I guess you don't take 'I can't,' 'I don't want to,' 'I don't feel like eating that,' or 'I hate grass' for an answer, do you?"

"Should I?" I asked.

"I hate it when you answer a question with a question."

"I know it hurts, but do you want to appear younger, feel healthier, and look slimmer?"

"Of course I do! Otherwise, why would I be wasting all this time with you?"

"Then let me suggest a strong, motivational tip."

"What is that?"

"Type this statement, 'I want to eat fruits and vegetables because I want to be healthy, so I love to eat fresh fruits and vegetables.'"

"What if I say that I don't know how to type?"

"You are lying, 'cause I know you can type! Otherwise, you would not have this job. You must have calluses on your fingertips spending eight hours a day beating up the laptop keyboards, and calling it a nursing job! At least, can you read your own handwriting?"

"Is that a question?"

"Good, 'cause I can't read mine. Otherwise I would have written it for you."

"Oh, very funny, Nik! Don't even get me started on your handwriting."

"Anyway, write this statement, 'I want to eat fruits and vegetables because I want to be healthy. So I love to eat fresh fruits and vegetables,' in your own handwriting, using bold letters, on a 3 x 5 card, and stick it onto the refrigerator on top of all those fast-food delivery coupons you have posted."

"How did you know that I have fast-food coupons on my refrigerator?"

"Well, I also used to. But that was before I learned of the benefits of including fresh fruits and vegetables in my daily dietary regimen."

"Now can you give me a shopping list so I don't have to walk around with your book in the grocery store, looking like a vegetable geek?"

"I can feel your pain, but do not despair. I have created a separate chart consisting of a list of carefully selected items. Just carry a copy of this in your handbag and keep it there until the ink turns illegible. Then, make another copy from the book to replace the old one. This will enable you to look like an intelligent, educated shopper."

"What do you mean by an intelligent, educated shopper? I shop alone most of the time. Are you suggesting that someone is watching me?"

"Of course, people are watching you all the time. Just because you are walking around with blinders over your eyes (and life) does not mean the world is not watching you. Let me ask you a question. If no one is watching you, why do you want to lose weight and look slim? Why are you listening to me?"

"Because I want to feel and look good for me."

"Then what is wrong with looking like an intelligent and educated shopper for yourself?"

"You are nuts!"

Well, I am giving you the nuts and bolts for a healthier, slimmer, younger-looking, and a heart-healthy lifestyle! You have to make up your mind if you want. Sitting in a church is not going to make you a Christian any more than sitting in a chicken house is going to make you a chicken."

"What do you mean?"

"People who just think and wish are a dime a dozen and those who put their ideas into practice are priceless."

"I didn't know that you attended a theological seminary."

"Common sense, Sandy! Common sense. That is what I have been trying to instill in your mind all this time. A well-balanced approach will go a long way in helping you achieve your desire."

"Enough, enough, get back to the main point, I don't have all day long."

"Well, when you meet one of your snobby friends, just unfold the long shopping list and make every effort to get their attention towards the shopping list."

"Why?"

"What are friends for? Show them that you know a lot more than most other people when it comes to grocery shopping. However, you do not want them to feel bad or inferior. Instead, you can use this opportunity to engage them in an uplifting, colorful, and intellectual conversation on how this shopping list has made a significant and positive change in your life. They will begin to pay attention and will be eager to know where you got that list. In the future, they may seek your advice on other Heart Healthy Lifestyle tips you have learned. Now you become an important resource for them. That should make you feel better about yourself and encourage you to stick with the Heart Healthy Lifestyle."

"Is this one of your advertising plots? Who gave you this idea?" Sandy asked.

"Believe me, it works. You might even make some new friends!"

"Get out of here!"

"Wait, I am not done. If you have a great idea, but you cannot share it with your family and friends, it is worthless!"

"What are you up to?"

"The next time you invite your friends and family over, keep a copy of the shopping list near your bar, cocktail tables, and the dining table. Let your guests soak up the list as they sip on a glass of red wine. Speaking of which, red wine also has antioxidants."

"Back to what you were saying, then what?"

"Serve them your antioxidant formulas for an appetizer — fresh fruits and vegetables."

"Are you out of your mind?"

Heart Healthy Choices
Fresh Fruits & Vegetables

Vegetables

Red bell peppers
Green bell peppers
Yellow bell peppers
Mushrooms
Zucchini
Romaine lettuce
Fresh spinach
Broccoli
Cauliflower
Asparagus
Cilantro
Cucumbers
Eggplant
Tomatoes

Beans

Kidney beans
Chickpeas
Peas
Soybeans

Fruits

Cantaloupe
Grapefruit
Strawberries
Blackberries
Blueberries
Raspberries
Strawberries
Olives
Peaches
Nectarines
Pears
Plums
Lemons
Oranges

Orange squash
Garlic

Nuts

Walnuts
Almonds
Hazelnuts

Fiber-Rich Diet

Fiber, an important part of a heart healthy diet, is not absorbed and passes through the digestive system largely intact. It is an essential part of our digestive process and it protects us against illnesses such as heart disease and cancer. Fiber is found only in plant foods, such as grains, fruits, vegetables, beans, nuts, and seeds.

What is fiber? Fiber is a complex carbohydrate that forms the supporting structure of fruits, vegetables, and grains (cellulose, hemi-cellulose, and lignans). There are two types of dietary fiber: soluble fiber that forms a gel when mixed with liquid and insoluble fiber that does not. The insoluble fiber is not digested by your digestive system and passes through the intestines unchanged. The soluble fibers are partially digested by the natural bacteria in the colon.

Why do you need dietary fiber? Fiber slows the absorption of fats and carbohydrates in your gastrointestinal tract, thus reducing the absorption of excess calories that can turn into body fat. It provides a sensation of fullness and suppresses your appetite by expanding to ten times its original size in your intestines.

Benefits of a High-Fiber Diet

Heart disease: A high dietary fiber intake has been demonstrated to lower the risk of heart disease in a number of large-scale studies. A Harvard study of over 40,000 male health professionals revealed that people on high-fiber diets had a 40% lower risk of coronary heart disease compared with those on a low-fiber diet. A related study of 68,000 women revealed similar results. Cereal fiber from grains seemed to be particularly beneficial. Diets especially high in soluble fiber have been shown to lower the total cholesterol by as much as 15 to 20 points.

Colon cancer: Relying on the results from a number of relatively small studies, for many years physicians have been advocating a high-fiber diet for lowering colon cancer risk. However, a Harvard study that followed over 80,000 female nurses for 16 years found that higher dietary fiber intake was not strongly associated with a reduced colon cancer risk.

Type 2 diabetes: Eating carbohydrates with a low glycemic index (GI) and adding fiber to your diet will slow the absorption of carbohydrates and reduce sudden insulin surges. Studies have shown that people who were on a high fiber diet had a 50% reduction in the development of type 2 diabetes. High GI foods such as potatoes, white bread, white rice, refined cereals (corn flakes, Cheerios), white spaghetti, and sugar should be used sparingly. Complement your daily diet with low GI foods such as whole fruits, oats, bran, beans, and whole-grain cereals.

Diverticular disease: Fiber has long been used in the prevention of diverticulitis, an inflammation of the colon pouches that is seen with increasing frequency with age. One-third of all Americans over age 45 and two-thirds of those over age 85 have symptoms of diverticular disease. The Harvard study of male health professionals found that people who were on a diet high in insoluble fiber had a 40% lower risk of diverticular disease.

Constipation: Constipation is one of the most common gastrointestinal complaints, particularly in the elderly population in the United States. Fiber increases bulk and facilitates intestinal motility, thus reducing symptoms of constipation. Wheat and oat bran fiber seem to be more effective in relieving constipation than fiber from fruits and vegetables. I recommend that you increase your fiber intake gradually and drink plenty of water, since the fiber absorbs a large amount of water.

While some research shows that a high-fiber diet may reduce the risk of obesity, high-fiber diets are not known for their weight loss advantages.

Fiber slows the absorption of calories from fats and carbohydrates. Fiber can expand 8 to 10 times its volume by absorbing water. This leads to increased bulk in the stomach, a sensation of fullness, and appetite suppression.

No harmful effects have been noted in people who have consumed Metamucil or Citrucel over a long time. In fact, these fiber products are routinely recommended for those with irritable bowel syndrome or diverticulitis. A diet in excess of 30 grams fiber may interfere with vitamin and mineral absorption.

How much fiber do you need? I recommend that you consume 20 to 30 grams of fiber per day. An average American diet provides only 5 to 7 grams. Try to incorporate fiber in your breakfast, lunch, and dinner. Addition of supplemental fiber also can boost your daily fiber intake.

What are the side effects? High-fiber diets can produce side effects such as nausea, diarrhea, and abdominal bloating. However, some of these symptoms may be minimized by gradually increasing your fiber intake over a several-week period.

What are good sources of dietary fiber? Start your day with a high-fiber breakfast cereal with 5 or more grams of fiber per serving. For example, half a cup serving of bran flake cereal has 5.5 grams and an unpeeled pear has 4.5 grams of fiber. Select cereals with the word bran or fiber in the name or add a few tablespoons of unprocessed wheat bran to your favorite cereal.

Oats, fruits, vegetables, and beans and peas are excellent sources of fiber for a high-fiber diet. Switch to whole-grain breads. Look for whole wheat, whole-wheat flour or another whole grain as the first ingredient on the label. Experiment with brown rice, barley, and whole-wheat pasta. Take advantage of today's ready-to-use vegetables. Beans, chickpeas, and lentils are good sources of fiber.

Fiber is an excellent choice for treatment of chronic constipation. However, if you experience acute constipation, consult with your physician, as it could be a sign of intestinal blockage.

Notes:

Chapter 08

Omega-3s Are Amazing
Essential fatty acids to watch

What Are Omega-3s?

Omega-3 fatty acids (omega-3s) are a form of polyunsaturated fatty acids, one of the four basic types of fat derived from food, along with cholesterol, saturated fat, and monounsaturated fat. Polyunsaturated fatty acids, including the omega-3s, have been shown to be important to human health.

Omega-3s are essential fatty acids, meaning your body cannot manufacture them. Therefore, they have to come from a dietary source. Omega-3s have an important role in maintaining the brain cells and in the arterial linings. An average American diet does not contain enough omega-3s to get the maximum benefit. You need to select special vegetables or seafoods that are rich in omega-3s or take supplements if you do not want to eat fish.

Classification of Omega-3s

All fatty acids contain carbon, oxygen, and hydrogen atoms. Fatty acids consist of a chain of hydrogen and carbon atoms (a hydrocarbon) that varies in length, with one acidic end. When every carbon atom has a hydrogen atom attached to it, the fat is saturated. Polyunsaturated fatty acids contain two or more double bonds (missing hydrogen atoms) in the middle of the chain. The omega nomenclature describes the position of the first double bond in the hydrocarbon chain.

All fatty acids compete for the same metabolic enzymes, resulting in alternating steps of removing hydrogen atoms (desaturation) and chain elongation. These metabolic steps occur only toward the acidic end of the molecule, keeping the first double bond from the other end the same. Mammals cannot insert a double bond at the third carbon position to produce omega-3s. They also cannot convert omega-6 fatty acids to omega-3s. Thus, both omega-6s and omega-3s must be supplied in the diet.

In omega-3s, the hydrogen atom on the third carbon atom is missing, creating a double bond between the third and fourth carbon atoms. The ability of the fatty acid chains to bend and stay in liquid form at very low temperatures depends on the number of missing hydrogen atoms. It's important for membranes in the cells to stay fluid at all temperatures, and that's controlled by fatty acid composition.

Omega-3s and related fatty acids are classified into different groups based on the number of hydrogen bonds and the length of the fatty acid chains:

- Alpha-linolenic acid (ALA)
- Eicosapentanoic acid (EPA)
- Docosahexaenoic acid (DHA)
- Gamma Linolenic acid (LA) (an Omega-6 fatty acid)

Alpha-linolenic acid (ALA): ALA has a double bond at the third carbon position (thus, the name omega-3, where omega refers to third position from the nonacidic end). Flaxseed oil (or capsules containing flaxseed oil) is a rich source of ALA. Dark green leafy vegetables and certain vegetable oils also contain ALA. Walnuts are another source of ALA. Your body has the ability to convert ALA to EPA. ALA acts as an anti-inflammatory agent, prevents arterial wall damage, and boosts your immune system.

Eicosapentaenoic acid (EPA): It is a major omega-3 fatty acid component of fish oil or deep-sea fish such as salmon, mackerel, rainbow trout, and tuna. EPA, being an important part of the brain cell membrane, maintains brain cells intact.

Docosahexaenoic acid (DHA): DHA is another omega-3, an important component of fish or fish oil, that maintains the integrity of the brain cell membrane. Since the human body cannot produce DHA, it has to come from a dietary source.

Linolenic acid (LA): This is an omega-6 essential fatty acid found in most vegetable oils (the double bond is at the sixth carbon). According to experts, our current consumption of this fatty acid has doubled from what it was in 1940. Excess intake of omega-6s increases water retention, raises blood pressure, and accelerates blood clotting.

Oleic acid (OA) is an omega-9 fatty acid. It is the predominant fatty acid seen in olive oil. Flaxseed contains a small percentage of this omega-9 fatty acid. Many other fats containing polyunsaturated fatty acids also contain oleic acid.

Role of Omega-3s

Cell membranes consist of two layers of phospholipids (a type of fat) and cholesterol with embedded proteins acting as hormone receptors, transporters, and enzymes. The phospholipid composition determines the physical and functional properties of cell membranes and has critical implications for cell integrity, growth, immunity, and anti-inflammatory properties.

Polyunsaturated fatty acids with twenty carbon atoms, found in cell membrane phospholipids, are precursors of eicosanoids. These eicosanoids include the prostaglandins, prostacyclins, and other hormones that control a variety of body functions, including blood pressure, health of blood vessels, regulating the white blood cells in the immune system, blood clotting, and cell division and cell differentiation.

Eicosanoids are also involved in stomach acid production, gastrointestinal motility, kidney blood flow, and salt excretion, as well as regulation of signals in the nervous system regulation, neuromuscular activity, and control of body temperature at the brain level.

Benefits of Omega-3s

A key clinical study, reviewing several long-term clinical trials, concluded that diets that included a regimen of increased omega-3s consistently showed a decrease in the cardiovascular disease incidence. These results were even better when compared to the results of other patients who were on a strict low-fat diet alone without supplemental omega-3s.

Neurological benefits: If someone says you have a fat brain, they are literally speaking the truth, because 60% of your brain is made up of fat. The brain cell membranes are rich in omega-3s. In reality, the omega-3s (especially the EPA and DHA) are believed to keep the brain's entire traffic pattern of thoughts, reactions, and reflexes running smoothly and efficiently. When the brain cannot get enough omega-3 fatty acids, it has to use other fatty acids that are not as flexible as the omega-3s. Replacement of omega-3s with less elastic fatty acids could lead to brain cell dysfunction. Adequate intake of omega-3s has been shown to reduce symptoms of depression, dementia, general anxiety, schizophrenia, and mood disorders. They also have been shown to improve cognitive and behavioral functions.

Stroke: Strong evidence from population-based studies suggests that omega-3s (mainly from fish) help protect against stroke caused by plaque buildup and blood clots in the arteries. Eating at least two servings of fish per week reduces the risk of stroke by as much as 50%. Nonetheless, people who eat more than 3 grams of omega-3s per day (equivalent to three servings of fish per day) may be at an increased risk for hemorrhagic stroke, a potentially fatal type of stroke in which a brain artery leaks or ruptures. However, the Alaskan Inuit (Eskimos), who consume as much as 14 grams of omega-3s per day, have not been shown to have an increased hemorrhagic stroke incidence. Therefore, it may be a combination of high omega-3s and other blood thinners that may increase such a risk, especially in the elderly population with weak arterial linings.

Infants: Omega-3s are vital for infants' health. Pregnant mothers who consume less omega-3s increase the potential risk of vision and nerve problems in their newborn babies.

Cardiovascular system benefits: Omega-3s lower blood cholesterol levels and also reduce arterial damage by their anti-inflammatory action. In addition, they lower the LDL (bad) cholesterol level, increase the HDL (good) cholesterol, and decrease platelet adhesiveness (that leads to clot formation). In the absence of polyunsaturated omega-3s, your body has to use saturated fats in its cell membranes, resulting in membranes that are less elastic, a situation that can have a negative effect on the heart muscle by making it harder to return to a relaxed state. Serious cardiac arrhythmias are also less common among people who consume large doses of omega-3s regularly. They also decrease the rate of plaque growth in the arterial lining.

Studies of heart attack survivors have found that daily omega-3 supplements dramatically reduce the risk of death, subsequent heart attacks, and stroke. Likewise, people who eat an ALA-rich diet are less likely to suffer a fatal heart attack.

High blood pressure: Large-scale studies have discovered that people who consume more omega-3s have lower blood pressure readings, as noted in Inuit, who consume oily cold-water fish. Avoid certain fish sources (such as tuna) that are high in mercury, since mercury is toxic and is known to increase blood pressure.

Immune system: Omega-3s seem to improve rheumatoid arthritis, diabetes, and psoriasis symptoms, as well as insulin sensitivity. They also have been shown to increase the life span of people with autoimmune diseases, because of their anti-inflammatory properties. The human body can convert EPA and DHA into natural anti-inflammatory substances called prostaglandins and leukotriene compounds that decrease inflammation and pain. People on high omega-3 diets have less joint stiffness, swelling, tenderness, and overall fatigue. They also need less pain medication.

Cancer: A recent study showed that participants who consumed fish oils as part of their diet produced lower quantities of carcinogens associated with colon cancer in comparison to those who were on a regular diet. There is increasing scientific evidence that omega-3s help preserve healthy breast tissue and prevent breast cancer.

The Mediterranean diet: This diet consists of a healthier balance between omega-3s and omega-6s. Many studies have shown that people who follow this diet are less likely to develop heart disease. The Mediterranean diet, which does not contain much meat (which is high in omega-6s), does comprise foods rich in omega-3s including whole grains, fresh fruits and vegetables, fish, olive oil, and garlic. This diet also includes moderate wine consumption.

Diabetes: People with diabetes tend to have high triglycerides and low HDL levels. Since omega-3s lower triglycerides and raise HDL, diabetic people may benefit from eating foods or taking supplements that contain EPA and DHA. However, ALA (an omega-3 from flaxseed) may not provide the same benefit as EPA or DHA, as some diabetic people lack the ability to efficiently convert ALA to the EPA or DHA that their body can readily use.

Weight loss: Omega-3s combined with low calories and low carbohydrates will improve insulin sensitivity and sugar control, aiding weight loss.

Osteoporosis: Omega-3s (such as EPA) increase the body and bone calcium levels, leading to improved bone strength. People deficient in EPA suffer from bone loss. A study in women over 65 with osteoporosis showed less bone loss and increased bone density over a three year period among those who received EPA and ALA supplements compared to those who did not.

Eating disorders: Men and women with anorexia nervosa have lower levels of polyunsaturated fatty acids (including ALA and GLA). To prevent the complications associated with essential fatty acid deficiencies, some experts recommend that treatment programs for anorexia nervosa patients should include ample supply of omega-3s in their diets.

Asthma: Omega-3 supplements (in the form of flaxseed oil, which is rich in ALA) may improve lung function in adults with asthma, due to its anti-inflammatory properties. In contrast, omega-6s (found in most vegetable oils) tend to increase inflammation and worsen respiratory function. In a small, well-designed study of twenty-nine children with asthma, those who took fish oil supplements (rich in EPA and DHA) for 10 months had improvement in their symptoms compared to those children who took a placebo (sugar) pill.

Inflammatory bowel disease (IBD): Omega-3s, when combined with a standard medication for IBD, such as sulfasalazine, may reduce symptoms of Crohn's disease and ulcerative colitis (two types of IBD). More studies exploring this preliminary finding are under way. In animals, it appears that ALA works better at decreasing bowel inflammation compared to EPA and DHA. However, the symptoms such as gas and diarrhea of IBD may also be caused by fish oil. Time-release preparations may help reduce these unwanted effects.

Burns: Essential fatty acids have been used to reduce inflammation and promote wound healing in burn victims. Omega-3s may promote a healthy balance of proteins in the body that is so vital for recovery after sustaining a burn.

Macular degeneration: Several studies have shown that people who regularly consumed omega-3s in the form of fish or fish oil capsules were less likely to have macular degeneration (a serious age-related eye condition that may lead to blindness) than those who consumed less fish. Another study confirmed this finding as well, in people who consumed fish (containing EPA and DHA) four or more times per week. In fact, the same study also noted that ALA might increase the risk of macular degeneration.

Menstrual pain: A Danish study showed that women with the highest dietary intake of omega-3s had the mildest symptoms during menstruation.

Colon cancer: Consuming significant amounts of omega-3s reduces the risk of colorectal cancer. For example, the Inuit, who follow a high fat diet but eat significant amounts of fish rich in omega-3 fatty acids, have a low rate of colorectal cancer. Daily consumption of EPA and DHA also slow or even reverse the progression of colon cancer in people with early stages of the disease.

Breast cancer: Although not all experts agree, women who regularly consume foods rich in omega-3s over many years may be less likely to develop breast cancer. In addition, the risk of dying from breast cancer may be significantly less for those who eat large quantities of omega-3 from fish and brown kelp seaweed (common in Japan). The balance between omega-3s and omega-6s appears to play an important role in the development and growth of breast cancer. Several researchers speculate that omega-3s in combination with other nutrients (namely, vitamin C, vitamin E, beta-carotene, selenium, and coenzyme Q10) may prove to be of particular value for preventing and treating breast cancer.

Prostrate cancer: Omega-3s (specifically, DHA and EPA) have been shown to inhibit the growth of prostate cancer in animal studies. Similarly, population-based studies of groups of men suggest that a low-fat diet with the addition of omega-3s from fish or fish oil helps prevent prostate cancer. Like breast cancer, the balance of omega-3 to omega-6 fatty acids appears to be particularly important for reducing the risk of this condition. ALA, however, may not offer the same benefits as EPA and DHA. In fact, one recent study evaluating 67 men with prostate cancer found that they had higher levels of ALA compared to men without prostate cancer. More research in this area is needed.

Daily Recommended Dose of Omega-3s

There is no established recommended daily intake for omega-3s. A healthy diet containing significant amounts of foods rich in these essential fatty acids is clearly wise. Experts believe that the ratio of the omega-6 fatty acids to omega-3 fatty acids must be 1:1. The average American diet has an omega-6 to omega-3 ratio in the range of 10:0 to 40:1. Do not fret. If you are reading this chapter, there is still some hope. Omega-6 fatty acids are present in such vegetable oils as olive oil, canola oil, and sunflower oil.

Pregnant women and infants need plenty of omega-3s to nourish the developing brain of the fetus and young child. If a pregnant woman's omega-3 fatty acid intake is too low, the growing fetus will take all that is available. This could set the stage for depression in the mother.

The American Heart Association recommends that people who have high triglycerides (blood fats) may benefit from a supplement of 2 to 4 grams of EPA and DHA per day.

Evidence from prevention studies suggests that taking a combination of EPA+DHA, ranging from 0.5 to 1.8 grams per day (either as fatty fish or supplements) significantly reduces deaths from heart disease, stroke, and all other causes. For ALA, a total intake of 1.5 to 3 grams per day seems beneficial.

Supplements also could help people with high triglycerides, who need even larger doses (2 to 4 grams per day).

Sources of Omega-3s

Aside from fresh seaweed, plant foods rarely contain EPA or DHA.

Increase your intake of fish such as salmon, mackerel, rainbow trout, or tuna, which are rich in omega-3 fatty acids. The American Heart Association recommends that people eat deep-sea fish such as salmon, mackerel, tuna or salmon at least twice a week.

Venison and buffalo are both good sources of omega-3s that make a healthy choice for people craving meat. These wild game meats can be purchased through mail-order sources if your supermarket does not carry them.

Omega-3 fatty acid supplements: You can take 3 to 4 grams standardized fish oils per day. This corresponds to 2 or 3 servings of deep-sea fatty fish such as salmon, mackerel, tuna, or trout per week. Please refer to the chart for details on other forms of fish that can provide omega-3 fatty acids. Typically, a 1000 mg fish oil capsule has 180 mg EPA and 120 mg DHA.

You can consume 6 capsules of fish oil per day, which will give you 1080 mg of EPA and 720 mg of DHA per day.

In raw flaxseed, 10 grams (2 tsp) provides 2.28 grams of ALA. Take at least two capsules of flaxseed oil. You can also buy fresh flaxseed oil in a bottle from Whole Foods Market or local nutritional stores. You cannot use flaxseed oil for cooking or seasoning, as heat will destroy its nutritional value. Instead, you can add flaxseed oil to already prepared foods or to your cereal. You can also add some to your salad and thus increase your intake of omega-3 fatty acids. Your body can convert the ALA from the flaxseed oil to EPA and DHA.

Essential fatty acids turn rancid and get bad very quickly. They should be kept away from light, heat, and air. they can last longer if kept in the fridge sealed well and in a dark bottle. Commercial processing also destroys them. Always buy fresh cold pressed. Finally, pesticides often gather in fats and oils, so buy organic products whenever possible.

Buy flaxseeds from Whole Foods Markets. You can get a pound of flaxseed for a few dollars. Use a teaspoon of flaxseeds in salads or cereals. You can also use a coffee grinder to grind the seeds to a fine powder and mix it into already prepared foods. It is better to grind only the amount you need at any given time. Keep the seeds in a refrigerator to prolong their shelf life.

Other vegetable sources include walnuts, pumpkin seeds, and leafy green vegetables. One ounce of walnuts supplies about 2 grams of plant-based omega-3 fatty acids, slightly more than that found in 3 ounces of salmon. However, seeds also have omega-6 fatty acids, which increase your calorie count. Therefore, you want to get those that have the highest amount of omega-3s per teaspoon of seeds.

Enhanced foods: In the U.S., these include omega-3 enriched eggs. However, beware of the fact that the cost of omega-3s enriched eggs may be two to three times that of ordinary eggs. You may be better off using supplemental fish oils, nuts, and seeds as described above.

People with either diabetes or schizophrenia may lack the ability to convert ALA to EPA and DHA, the forms that are readily taken up by the brain cells. Therefore, people with these conditions should obtain their omega-3s from dietary sources rich in EPA and DHA.

Cholesterol-lowering medications: Following certain nutritional guidelines, including increasing the amount of omega-3s in your diet and reducing the omega-6 to omega-3 ratio, may allow a group of cholesterol lowering medications known as statins such as Lipitor to work more effectively.

Precautions: Omega-3s reduce platelets' stickiness, which can lead to bleeding problems in patients who are already on any blood thinners such as aspirin, Coumadin, or other antiplatelet agents. If you are taking more than 3 grams of omega-3 supplements, do so only with your physician's supervision. High intake could cause excessive bleeding in some people.

Fish oil capsules may leave a fishy taste or may cause burping. However, it's not so bad that everyone in the room will have to leave. You will learn to live with it. In due course, you may forget about it or not even notice when it occurs.

Certain older, larger predatory fish may contain high levels of mercury, PCBs (polychlorinated biphenyls), dioxins, and other environmental contaminants. Eating a variety of fishes will help minimize any potentially adverse effects due to environmental pollutants.

From a caloric viewpoint, all oils are equally fattening. They contain 120 calories per tablespoon. Fish oil can cause gas and diarrhea. Time-release preparations may reduce these side effects.

Omega-3s should be an important part of our daily diet. Make sure you get 2 to 4 grams of omega-3s from various sources such as seafood, oils, and nuts.

Heart Healthy Lifestyle

Omega-3 Contents of Various Foods (in grams)

Deep-sea fish	O-6s	O-3s	LNA	EPA	DHA
Mackerel	1.1	2.2	0.1	0.9	1.6
Herrings	0.6	1.7	0.1	1.0	0.7
Sardines		1.7			
Bluefin tuna		1.7	--	0.4	1.2
Trout		1.7			
Salmon (Atlantic)	0.7	1.4	0.2	0.3	0.9
Anchovies		1.4			
Bluefish	0.4	1.3	--	0.4	0.8
Halibut	0.5	0.9	Tr	0.5	0.4
Rainbow trout		0.8			
Bass, striped	--	0.8	Tr	0.2	0.6
Shrimp	0.2	0.4	Tr	0.2	0.1
Catfish	0.7	-	Tr	0.1	0.2
Sturgeon	0.6	-	Tr	1.0	0.5
Conch	0.1	-	Tr	0.6	0.4

Oils, 100 g					
Flaxseed oil			15.0	58	-
Walnut oil			58.0	11.5	-
Canola oil			20.0	7.0	11.2
Soybean oil			51.0	7.0	-
Hazelnuts			4.0	Tr	-
Cashews			8.0	Tr	-
Butter			1.8	1.2	-

Seeds, 100 g					
Flaxseeds			6.0	15-25	-
Pumpkin seeds			20.0	7-10	-
Sunflower seeds			30.0	Tr	-
Walnuts			34.2	3.3	-
Soybean kernels			11.2	1.5	-

Tr = trace; – none detectable

Chapter 09

Drinks & Caffeine
Water is not a stimulant

Drinks

The next time you order a drink, think twice. What is in that drink? This article will shed some light on the most commonly ordered drinks, their composition, and the myths behind their labels. A common recipe for a drink is sugar, caffeine, alcohol, a mystery ingredient, and tap water.

Soda: Most sodas have water, sugar, and a brand-name secret ingredient. An average 12-ounce can of soda has 150 calories, 35 grams of sugar (9 teaspoons!), 60 to 100 mg of caffeine, and water. A 12-ounce can of Sunkist has 190 calories and 52 grams of sugar.

Beer: A twelve-ounce can of a typical beer has 150 calories, and 30 grams of alcohol. A light beer has approximately 90 to 120 calories. If you are drinking beer because you are thirsty, think again. Alcohol acts as a diuretic. It makes you lose more water than you get with your beer. If you sit and have four bottles of beer, you added 600 calories. That is just from your happy hour drink alone! A 12-ounce can of Sierra Nevada Stout has 210 calories.

Energy drinks: Do not be fooled by the drinks that are labeled "energy drinks." Even your regular soda is an energy drink. Energy in drinks comes mostly from carbohydrates or alcohol, and not from some secret ingredient. You may feel high or excited from an energy drink because of stimulants in the form of caffeine. A 12-ounce can of Rockstar Original has 280 calories and 68 grams of sugar.

If sugar makes you high, then you are addicted to sugar just like someone can be addicted to alcohol or cigarettes. It is time for you to join a sugar anonymous group or start one for you and your buddies.

Coffee: Many people have developed a taste for coffee, not knowing what they are getting. The alertness that you get from drinking a cup of coffee comes from caffeine, a natural stimulant found in coffee, and also added to many other products, including cold medicine. An average cup of coffee has 60 to 80 mg of caffeine. The calories come from sugar added to the coffee. So, a simple coffee may contain 8 ounces of hot water, 5 to 10 grams of sugar, some fat from milk, and 60 to 80 mg of caffeine, which is not bad. However, coffee drinks may give you more than you asked for. For example, a Starbucks Venti Peppermint White Chocolate Mocha made with 2% milk has a whopping 660 calories, 22 grams of fat (14 grams of saturated fat) and 95 grams of sugar.

A frozen coffee drink such as a Cosi Double Oh! Arctic-Gigante (24 ounce) has 1003 calories, 35 grams of fat, 177 grams of carbo-hydrates, 12 grams of protein, and 511 mg of sodium. It pays to read labels.

Tea: Just like coffee, tea also contains caffeine. Some claim that green tea has antioxidants. As long as you are drinking a cup of black or white tea, it is all right. But, when you start adding 3 to 4 teaspoons of sugar and 4 to 5 servings of Half & Half, you are asking for trouble. When you start ordering some fancy tea combinations, then you are talking about some big calories and unwanted fat. For example, a Caribou Coffee Large Chai Tea Latte has 420 calories and 47 grams of sugar.

Beware of iced tea in a can. It can be loaded with lots of sugar. A 20-ounce bottle of Lipton Brisk Iced Tea has 210 calories and 55 grams of sugar!

Diet drinks: You are calorie conscious and you want to switch to a diet drink. It's a good start. But, I want you to think a little more. Your diet drinks still may have caffeine. If you drink 4 to 5 cans of a diet drink containing caffeine, you are still getting that excess amount of caffeine. A better approach would be to have a diet drink which has no caffeine. If you can live without the calories and caffeine, then you might as well fill your plastic bottle and tap water and label it, "Nik's Diet Drink"! No, you don't have to use my name. You can put your spouse's name and make that person immensely happy. OK! It is just a suggestion.

Lemonade: What could possibly be wrong with a glass of lemonade? Sure, it's a good drink if it contains water, lemon juice and a sweetener. When the sweetener happens to 30 to 50 grams of sugar, Houston, we've got a problem! A 20-ounce bottle of Minute Maid Lemonade has 250 calories and 68 grams of sugar.

The next time you visit a restaurant, ask for a few slices of lemon. Most of the time, you can get it, compliments of the chef. Squeeze the lemon juice in a glass of ice water. Add a packet of sweetener. Now, you have a zero-calorie lemonade. Don't share this information with your waiter. The waiter may label you as a freeloader, and start charging you.

Smoothie: If you are ordering fruit juice as a smoothie, you are in for a surprise. Most fruits have fructose, which is a form of sugar. So, you will get your share of sugar in a fruit flavor. A 30-ounce Large Peanut Butter Moo'd Smoothie from Jamba Juice loads 1170 calories, 30 grams of fat, 192 grams of carbs, and 35 grams of protein. That is almost a day's worth of food. Unless you are trying to put on some weight before your wedding reception, you may want to stay away from such drinks.

Milk shakes: What is in a milk shake? It has milk with protein, sugar, fat, calcium, and sodium. If you are an adult, you do not need all that extra sugar and fat. Take, for example, a basic milk shake, which has 328 calories, 50 grams of carbohydrates, 7 grams of fat, and 18 grams of protein. However, as you move to more commercial brands, the calorie counts mount. For example, Denny's 12-ounce vanilla milk shake has 560 calories, 26 grams of fat, 76 grams of carbohydrates, and 11 grams of protein. Compare that with 8 ounces of skim milk, which has 80 calories, 7 grams of protein, zero grams of fat, and 11 grams of carbohydrates.

A Baskin-Robbins 24-ounce chocolate milk shake has 990 calories, 40 grams of fat, 149 grams of carbohydrates, and 20 grams of protein. You have to jog for 2 hours to burn those calories!

Water: Water by any other name is an expensive imitation. Do not be enticed into thinking a special mineral water is better than regular water. Your body needs 8 glasses of water per day. The best choice is to get tap water or bottled water. There is no advantage in spring water or water from other sources, or even among brands. In fact, several bottling companies use regular water to fill their labeled bottles. Yes, the tap water may contain impurities such as unwanted minerals and organic matter, among others. It also contains chlorine used as a disinfectant. Some people have put a water purifying filter between the main water line and the line coming in to the kitchen. If you can afford to do that, it is fine. You can live without extra sugar, excess calories, and caffeine. But, you cannot live without water. So make sure that you get at least 8 glasses of water per day.

Final tips: If you are not sure what the composition of your favorite drink is, visit the supplier's website and look for the caloric information. Most fast-food restaurants have posted the composition and calorie counts on their websites. Most cans have their ingredients printed on the cans. You can also visit your local bookstore and spend a Sunday evening browsing through a calorie count book to get a firsthand look at the composition of various drinks and make an educated decision about the next drink you want to order.

I do not want you to think I'm cynical about all drinks. But, it pays to know what is in the drink that you order. I'm trying to help you to become an educated consumer.

If you are eating a healthy diet, you can live a better life without that added sugar, excess caffeine, alcohol, vitamins, and minerals. The only useful ingredient in any drink is water and you might as well carry a bottle of tap water (certified by your city health department to be safe) and live a healthier life.

Caffeine & Its Cardiac Effects

Some time ago, while I was taking history from an 83-year-old lady, I asked, "Ma'am, do you drink coffee?"

"Yes," she said.

"How many cups?" I continued.

"Five cups a day, Doc," she replied.

"Ma'am, do you realize that coffee is a slow poison?" I pressed.

"It must be, Doc. I'm 83 years old and it's still trying to get me!"

Is coffee getting on your nerves? You are not alone. More importantly, it also seems to be having an impact on your credit cards, too!

An estimated 85 million people consume caffeine in the form of coffee, tea, chocolate, sodas, and some nuts. Americans seem to have a love affair with coffee. The more expensive the coffee, the better they feel! The more caffeine, the merrier they feel! That's where the real problems begin. Caffeine is a drug with notable cardiovascular and central nervous system effects which can last way beyond your last cup of coffee.

Caffeine dose: A regular cup of coffee (8 ounces) has approximately 50 to 60 mg of caffeine. Brewed coffee can contain as much as 115 mg of caffeine. Soft drinks containing caffeine have roughly 20 to 65 mg of caffeine per 12-ounce can. The FDA has recommended a limit of 68 mg caffeine per drink. However, some energy drinks may have caffeine well above the FDA recommended doses. Twelve ounces of iced tea contains 70 mg of caffeine. Starbucks Doubleshot has more than 105 mg and SoBe No Fear has as much as 141 mg per 16-ounce drink. Daily caffeine consumption should be less than 300 mg, or equivalent to less than 3 drinks per day.

Extra-strong caffeine tablets containing as much as 200 mg of caffeine are sold on the market and are sometimes used by athletes. Caffeine is also found in some medicines such as Exedrin, Midol, No-Doz, etc. Consuming more than 250 mg of caffeine at one time can cause a person to develop symptoms of caffeine intoxication, which are exaggerated central nervous system symptoms.

Caffeine effects: Caffeine belongs to a group of chemicals similar to the theophylline used to relieve bronchospasm in asthma patients. It is a central nervous system stimulant. Caffeine is normally metabolized and excreted in the urine within a few hours. The effects of caffeine last only a few hours.

It raises blood pressure. However, the temporary rise in blood pressure does not lead to chronic hypertension (long-standing high blood pressure). People who drink more than 5 cups of coffee per day have double the risk of heart disease compared with those who do not drink coffee. It can also increase heart rate and cause palpitations. Coffee, especially boiled and processed at high temperatures (like espresso), has been known to increase total cholesterol and LDL cholesterol levels. Coffee also elevates the levels of an amino acid in the blood called homocysteine. Elevated homocysteine has been associated with increased risk of heart disease. Caffeine also increases the adrenaline and cortisol (stress hormone) levels in the blood. However, some studies have shown a reduced risk of heart disease symptoms in people over 65 who consume caffeine containing drinks compared with younger populations.

Caffeine interferes with sleep, especially if you drink caffeine containing drinks late in the evening or at night. Did you ever wonder why you couldn't sleep after you had a regular soda late in the evening or in the middle of the night?

Caffeine has other effects on the nervous system. It makes kids hyperactive. In most people, it can cause the hands to shake.

It also releases free fatty acids from the fatty tissue. It increases urination which can lead to dehydration. In addition, there is increased loss of magnesium and calcium in the urine. There is no correlation between moderate caffeine consumption and cancer. It increases acid production in the stomach. However, caffeine does not help in weight loss. Exercise does!

Caffeine withdrawal: Caffeine is habit-forming. People who are used to regular caffeine consumption experience withdrawal symptoms 12 hours after their last dose of caffeine. They may have headache, anxiety, nervousness, fatigue, drowsiness, and depression. If you are trying to kick the caffeine habit, take a little time. Your body needs to get adjusted over time. Some people may be able to quit cold turkey, just as someone would try for smoking cessation or alcohol withdrawal. However, you may try reducing your coffee intake week by week and then eliminate it totally. Replace regular coffee with decaffeinated drinks to reduce caffeine dependence.

Management: Moderation is the key when it comes to caffein-ated drink consumption. Having 2 to 3 cups of caffeine containing drinks per day has not been associated with serious illnesses. Preg-nant women are encouraged to keep their caffeine intake to less than 120 mg, or less than 2 drinks per day.

If you are having significant symptoms related to caffeine, you should seriously consider reducing or eliminating the caffeine habit. First, begin by getting rid of caffeinated soft drinks. Replace your so-das with plain water. Second, you may consider caffeine-free drinks in place of drinks that contain caffeine. Decaffeinated drinks reduce the adrenaline rush and central nervous system symptoms, but they do not reduce the heart disease risk. Avoid caffeinated drinks in the evening if you are taking a test or have a mission-critical job the next morning in order to avoid sleeping through your test or job.

Energy drinks may seem to give you a boost which results from large doses of sugar and high levels of caffeine. You may consider regular sleep, good exercise, and healthy eating habits as a safer means to get energy.

Notes:

Chapter 10

Breakfast & Lunch

Breakfast

Tina, a young high school senior with heart palpitations, came to my office with her mom.

"Hi, I am Dr. Nikam. How can I help you?" I said.

"For the past few days at school, I've noticed my heart fluttering along with dizziness and weakness," she said.

"Did you ever pass out?" I asked.

"No."

"Do you ever get chest pains?"

"Sometimes. I have heaviness in the left side of my chest. It feels uncomfortable."

"Do you play any sport?" I quizzed.

"That's the thing I can't understand," her mom interjected. "In the afternoons when she's active during gymnastics and cheerleading, she's fine."

"That's a lot of exercise," I sighed.

"Do you get the same symptoms when you are actively involved in your activities?"

"No!"

"Honey, sometimes you had chest pain when you were running," her mother interjected again.

"Mom! That was when I was pushing myself too hard. Not anymore."

"Tina, do you eat breakfast?" I continued.

"In the morning I'm not hungry."

"Do you eat breakfast?" I repeated.

"You see, I'm always in a hurry, I don't have time."

"If you were not in a hurry, would you eat breakfast?"

"Well, probably not."

"Why not?" I said.

"'Cause I never eat breakfast."

"What if someone makes you breakfast?"

"If I'm not in the mood, ah, no," she said.

"Those are all the questions I have for you," I concluded. "Now, let me go ahead and check your heart."

I did a complete cardiac workup on Tina: physical examination, EKG, echocardiogram, and a 24 hour heart monitor, along with thyroid, blood sugar, and other blood tests. Everything came out satisfactory, except for one test. At the end of a three-hour glucose tolerance test, her blood sugar level was 61 mg. When someone's blood sugar level drops below 80 mg, they are known to have hypoglycemia—low blood sugar. Tina's case illustrates the importance of eating breakfast to maintain the steady blood sugar level needed for optimal performance.

The maximum daily demands on your body are during the early morning hours. That is when you need to have a readily available balanced energy source. Proper hydration is equally important, which I I addressed earlier in the "Drinks" chapter. In the morning hours, both children and adults have shown better concentration, performance, and muscle coordination, when their energy levels are optimal.

During the night, your body mainly depends on fat for a constant energy source. After 10 to 12 hours of fasting during the night, your blood glucose levels are generally low in the early morning hours, as was the situation in Tina's case. Activities such as walking, talking, showering, cursing, and rushing to work or school place extra demands on your body for a fresh supply of energy.

Critical learning, coordination, and physical activities require a readily available source of glucose, which is much easier for the muscle and brain tissues to utilize than fatty acids. In addition to glucose, you also need other macro- and micronutrients in the morning, which I will discuss shortly in this chapter.

Benefits of Eating Breakfast

Let us look at the benefits of having breakfast regularly, including holidays and weekends.

- Breakfast provides a fresh supply of energy for increased metabolic demands in the early hours of the morning.
- It improves learning.
- It increases your ability to focus.
- It improves muscle coordination.
- It supplies calories, protein, fat, and essential nutrients.
- It also provides vitamins, minerals, and fiber.
- It helps to evenly distribute your calories throughout the day.
- People who eat breakfast are less irritable than those who skip breakfast.
- It reduces the need for snacks or carbohydrate binges be tween your meals.

Lame excuses do not solve the problems that we face in the morning hours. It takes less than five minutes to eat your breakfast, and it takes less than thirty seconds to drink a glass of skim milk.

After several hours of fasting, everyone's blood sugar level may not drop to the level we saw in Tina's case. In fact, some people have fasted for sixty to ninety days without significant adverse effects. Each person's metabolism is different. A small percentage of people may not have noticeable cardiovascular symptoms related to hypoglycemia. On the other hand, dehydration, stress, or anxiety can precipitate symptoms of weakness, dizziness, and lack of energy in the absence of hypoglycemia. These factors underscore the importance of proper hydration and control of stress or anxiety during the challenging hours of your day.

During a severely stressful situation, the body responds by releasing adrenaline, which increases the blood glucose level by breaking down glycogen and by converting amino acids to glucose for immediate energy needs. Adrenaline also causes significant palpitations, weakness, dizziness, or flushing. The key to avoiding adrenaline surges and its symptoms is to maintain proper hydration and calorie intake, and reduce stress.

What Type of Breakfast Is Heart Healthy?

A suitable breakfast should include complex carbohydrates, proteins, minerals, vitamins, water, and fiber. You can get these components from dairy products, cereals, breads, and fruits. Let us look some of these food products and their composition.

Skim milk: The best breakfast in town or out of town (if you are on the run). It is an excellent source of protein and low glycemic index (GI) carbohydrates. One carton (8 ounces of milk) has 8 grams of protein, 11 grams of carbs, calcium, zero fat, and 80 calories. Look for calcium-fortified skim milk, which provides additional calcium. If you do not like to drink plain skim milk, consider making your coffee or tea using skim milk. You get three for the price of one—coffee, fluid, and milk.

Sugar: Substitute your table sugar with a sweetener—Equal or Splenda—and further reduce your carbohydrate intake. I have seen, in doctors' dining rooms, some of my friends putting 3 to 4 packets of pure sugar in their drinks, as well as 3 to 6 servings of Half & Half—bless their hearts!

Juices: Fresh fruits are a preferred choice over fruit juices. Fruits contain minerals, fibers, enzymes, and vitamins. They also do not have the preservatives or extra sugar added for taste. Remember, fruits or fruit juices contain carbohydrates and add extra calories to your diet.

Eggs: They are an excellent source of readily digestible protein (albumin). However, a single egg contains 274 mg of cholesterol, besides fat. The American Heart Association recommends no more than 300 mg of cholesterol per day. If you eat a three-whole-egg breakfast, then you get more than 800 mg of cholesterol—that, too, at the crack of dawn. Protein is good; but 800 mg of cholesterol is not. You have a couple of options. You can use an egg substitute that has no cholesterol. It comes as a yellow liquid in cartons. You also can use that to make omelets or scrambled eggs. The second option is to use egg white and discard the yolk. My friends think I am crazy to throw away the best part of the egg. Well! They have a point when it comes to taste and texture. However, they will not be there to cheer you up when the same cholesterol clogs up your arteries. A three-egg-white omelet can provide you 10 grams of protein and zero cholesterol! You also can prepare your egg-white omelets in a microwave. Pour two or three egg whites on a flat plate and cook them in a microwave for 45 to 75 seconds. You get a nice fluffy egg-white omelet. You can add your favorite spices, salt, onions, bell pepper, soybean sausage, or other ingredients to make it more palatable.

Sausage and bacon: Even though these breakfast items are favored in certain diets, they contain a high percentage of saturated fat. For example, a sausage patty contains 12 g of fat. As an alternative, you could try low-fat turkey sausage or bacon or soy sausage or bacon.

Cereals: Contrary to the conventional wisdom that cereals are good—not all cereals are created equal. There are a lot of bad cereals and a few good ones. Putting a celebrity picture on a box does not make a cereal heart healthy. If you carefully read the labels on the cereals, you will realize that most of them have 25 to 30 grams of high glycemic index (GI) carbohydrates. Some of them have visible sugar or sugar icing on them to entice your appetite. I can understand the marketing gimmick used by advertising agencies to allure working mothers to reach out for a quick-fix cereal breakfast to get the kid on the road again. However, a reality check should begin at home and with working mothers. Remember that your options are limited by the choices that are stocked in your kitchen. Therefore, if you cultivate a heart-healthy habit, it is bound to spill over to the next generation.

Cereals heavily promoted as crispy, tasty, or zesty, are high in sugars and high GI carbohydrates. Nevertheless, it is your mission to select 20 to 30 grams of carbohydrates for breakfast from the low

GI list that maintains your blood glucose levels over a longer period. Due to pressure from the consumer industry, the cereal manufacturers are slowly responding by bringing more heart-healthy cereals—Fiber One, All-Bran, Kashi—all of which have less carbohydrate, more fiber, and even cholesterol reducing properties. These cereals are welcome to someone concerned about a Heart Healthy Lifestyle. Don't forget to use the skim milk with your cereals.

Hydration: Keeping hydrated is very important after fasting for 10 to 12 hours, as your body loses water in urine, perspiration and metabolism (insensible losses). Hence, hydration should be an essential part of your breakfast regimen. I recommend Metamucil to all my cardiac patients. It helps to hold water in the body for several hours, in addition to its cholesterol lowering properties. I take it personally. Take one tablespoon of Metamucil along with two to three glasses of water. Then use another glass of water for your vitamins, aspirin, fish oil, flaxseed capsules, etc. Add to that a glass of skim milk in your coffee or tea. Now, even before you leave your house, you are well hydrated with four to five glasses of fluids. If you are well hydrated, you are less likely to have your blood pressure drop or to feel dizzy when there is a sudden adrenaline surge leading to dilation of the blood vessels. It may also minimize palpitations, weakness, and nausea or queasy feeling in your stomach.

Restaurant breakfast tips: Fast food restaurants are not interested in calories, carbohydrates, or fat content. It is up to you to choose food items that are likely to promote a Heart Healthy Lifestyle.

Let us analyze a sample breakfast menu from a fast food restaurant. Pancakes and hash browns are loaded with high GI carbohydrates. We talked about the cholesterol in an omelet made from three whole eggs. Do not let the looks deceive you. This breakfast is a mixture of saturated fat, cholesterol, carbohydrates, and no fiber.

"There are not too many choices." These are common complaints I hear from people whose lives revolve around restaurant menus. You do not need many choices. Just stop making the wrong choices based on an impulse, peer pressure, taste, or path of least resistance.

Look for skim milk, Egg Beaters, high fiber cereals, fresh fruits, simulated bacon, non-sugar sweeteners, or plain water. These choices should be enough to get you through the restaurant temptations.

When you're cruising across a breakfast buffet, remember that it's not how much you're paying for the buffet, but how much you'll have to pay to unclog your heart arteries in the future, and how much pain, grief, and loss of work you have to endure.

Breakfast choices: Here is a partial list of the heart healthy breakfast items that you could consider:

- Skim milk
- Egg white or substitutes
- Simulated bacon or sausage
- Vegetable or turkey sausage
- High-fiber cereals such as Fiber One, All-Bran, Kashi, etc.
- Small plain bagel
- Benecol (lowers cholesterol) instead of margarine
- Fresh fruits instead of sweetened juices
- Coffee or tea
- Non-sugar sweetener in place of sugar
- Fiber-rich, low-calorie, and protein-rich whole wheat bread
- Soy sausage links and patties
- Non-fat yogurt
- Fat-free cottage cheese
- One pancake with minimal syrup
- Low-fat Canadian bacon

Cooking tips: We routinely cook egg white or egg substitute in a microwave. Place the egg white in a cereal bowl and cook it in a microwave for 60 to 90 seconds. It will result in a nice fluffy blend. You also can add spices, onion, and bell pepper for taste.

- Cook a bagel in a toaster oven and add Benecol, a source of plant sterols and stanols that lower blood cholesterol levels.

- Consider adding a tablespoon of flaxseeds to your cold cereal to increase your omega-3 intake.
- Make your coffee or tea using skim milk so you do not need to add Half & Half.
- Select high-fiber, low-calorie, and high protein whole wheat bread in place of white bread.
- Avoid cereals rich in high GI carbohydrates.
- Avoid croissants (300 calories) or muffins (400 calories) that are high in carbohydrates, fats, and calories.

Nik's Breakfast Burrito:

If you can prepare Nik's burritos using just plain egg white or egg substitute, it can provide you a very nutritious breakfast without the extra cholesterol that you get with regular eggs.

You need the following ingredients:

- Chopped onions
- Chopped bell pepper
- Can of unsalted mushrooms, chopped
- One to two teaspoons of olive oil
- Two cartons of Egg Beaters
- Two soybean sausage patties
- Salt, pepper, or your favorite choice of spices
- One diced tomato
- Fiber-rich small tortillas

Put the olive oil in a medium sized pan. Mix all the chopped ingredients including onions, bell pepper, and mushrooms, and let them cook for three to five minutes. Cook the sausage patties in a microwave for at least forty-five seconds to one minute on each side, then crumble them. Add the egg and crumbled sausage patties to the pan. Stir the mixture until the Egg Beaters are dry and scrambled.

Toast a small high-fiber tortilla in a toaster oven. Now you can take a small portion of the scrambled egg mixture and wrap it with the tortilla to create Nik's Burrito. You can put the remaining scrambled egg mixture into small Ziploc bags and put them in the freezer for future use.

As you can see, I have carefully researched all the items that are available in the breakfast section of a supermarket. Then, I have selected those items that are rich in proteins, low in carbohydrates, fat, and cholesterol and high in fiber content. I have also taken into account the minerals and the micronutrients that you can get from fresh fruits and vegetables.

Lunch—On the Work Bench

As the title suggests, most people have their lunches on their work benches, unless you are an executive used to two hour lunch meetings at a gourmet restaurant. Therefore, let us get some understanding of lunch options. A basic lunch consists mostly of sandwiches, drinks, and desserts.

Drinks: Let's start with the drinks. Water is the most important drink you need during lunch. You can avoid the regular sodas that have 150 to 200 calories and 30 to 50 grams of carbohydrates. Most places you can get water for free, while you may have to pay money to get a soft drink. Even if you get a diet drink, keep in mind that most of them have caffeine, unless you buy a diet, caffeine-free drink. Then why would you want to spend money for a drink that has nothing? Get plain water. It is free in most cafeterias. A plain glass of water is fine. You can handle the minerals in the tap water.

Here is an idea you can try. Get a glass of water. Squeeze two slices of lemon, which you can get it for free. Add a sweetener of your choice. Now, you have your brand of soft drink. Don't tell anyone. You could also consider a carton of milk that can provide extra protein, calcium and minerals.

Lunch proteins: Lunchmeats are an excellent source of protein with minimal fat. Each slice has 1 ounce of meat with 8 to 12 grams of high-quality protein. You can use 2 to 3 slices to provide you with

15 to 20 grams of good protein. Combine your salads and fruits with your lunchmeat and you have one of the best lightweight heart healthy lunches that you can carry with you wherever you go. Look for meats that are fat-free, which further reduces the calorie intake.

Here is a partial list of lunch choices:

- Grilled chicken breast—Cajun, lime pepper
- Turkey sandwich
- Four ounces of grilled salmon
- Chick peas
- Beans
- Turkey burger without bun
- Salsa
- Salad with light dressing
- Cottage cheese
- Sandwiches with low-calorie wheat bread and low-fat cheese
- Veggie burger

Lunch carbs: It is very easy to fill up with carbs before you know it. Consider the bread served as an appetizer along with butter. The breadsticks, croutons, pasta, rice, potato chips, mashed potatoes, and the list goes on and on. French fries, chips, and nachos are a combination of both carbs and fat. Try to keep your carb intake to a minimum. If you do pick a chip packet, try to share it with your colleagues so that you are not filling up with 200 to 400 empty calories. A bag of potato chips may have 210 calories, with 30 grams of carbs and 9 grams of fat. A large tortilla may have as much as 300 to 400 calories, most of it coming from carbs.

Salads: If you are not accustomed to routine salads, consider eating salad 2 to 3 times per week. This will help to balance out your excess calorie intake during the evening or weekends. I have seen people who can pack more than 1000 calories with their salad itself. Here are some simple tips in loading up your salad plate. Fill it up with romaine lettuce or your favorite choice. Add carrots, bell peppers, tomatoes, mushrooms, cottage cheese, olives, and grilled chicken pieces. Skip the bacon, baked potatoes, and croutons. Save the breads for a later afternoon snack. You are done. No, wait. I just forgot, you have to add a tablespoon of flaxseeds. Yes, flaxseeds are rich in omega-3s. Now, you are done. You may ask, "What about the dressing?" The cows don't use any dressing. You do not need two ounces of dressing, which can add 500 to 600 calories. I learned to eat the salad with no dressing. If you insist, you could take some olive oil in a small cup on the side and dip your salad on the way to your lips.

Nik's Burger: Yes, indeed, you can have hamburger meat provided you follow these steps. A regular hamburger patty may have more than 50% of its weight as fats, and contribute to more than 70% of the calories. In addition, it also has a high percentage of saturated fats. Take, for example, 7% fat ground turkey. Sounds good, doesn't it, only 7% fat? However, when you count the calories, you will be surprised to find out that 50% of the calories are coming from fat sources. Ostrich meat has 3% fat by weight. Please note that water makes up 80% of the meat weight. You can also try chicken burgers, which have lower amounts of fat and calories.

If you must have a hamburger, here are some useful tips. Try a veggie burger. Always use small buns and double up on the veggie patties if you want. Add lots of tomatoes, onions, and lettuce to pile up your burger. Avoid using mayonnaise. Instead, add nothing. Also avoid toasting your bread with butter—another source of saturated fat. Instead, select whole-wheat bread and toast it in an oven or over a grill. Add a little lemon and pepper to give some taste to your burger. Alternatively, you could replace your French fries with salsa. The fast food restaurants may be offended by these recommendations, but that is all right. I am the one who is interested in your Heart Healthy Lifestyle, not them. For drinks, have a glass of water with a little lemon juice and a sweetener. That is a zero calorie drink. So you can indeed enjoy a hamburger that is less than 300 calories compared with a 1500 calorie Double Whopper burger lunch at a fast food joint.

Desserts: Just say no! Lunch time is not the best time for a mouth-watering dessert. You can save that for the evening dinner.

Consider some fruit that won't put you to sleep on the job.

Breakfast Choices: Checklist

- Skim milk
- Egg white or substitutes
- Simulated bacon or sausage
- Vegetable or turkey sausage
- High-fiber cereals such as Fiber One, All-Bran, Kashi, etc.
- Small plain bagel
- Benecol (lowers cholesterol) instead of margarine
- Fresh fruits instead of sweetened juices
- Coffee or tea
- Non-sugar sweetener in place of sugar
- Fiber-rich, low-calorie, and protein-rich whole wheat bread
- Soy sausage links and patties
- Non-fat yogurt
- Fat-free cottage cheese
- One pancake with minimal syrup
- Low-fat Canadian bacon

Lunch Options:

- Grilled chicken breast—Cajun, lime pepper
- Turkey sandwich
- Four ounces of grilled salmon
- Chick peas
- Beans
- Turkey burger without bun
- Salsa
- Salad with light dressing or no dressing
- Cottage cheese
- Sandwiches with low-calorie wheat bread and low-fat cheese.
- Veggie burger
- Water

Chapter 11

Everyday Dinner
Makes life more enchanting

The other day, Sonia asked me if I could write an article for Valentine's Day, talking about foods that accent a romantic theme.

"How about a nice chicken biryani or lamb curry?" I asked.

She said, "No, not that routine stuff. It has to appeal and leave a memorable experience."

"Oh! You mean something novel for the take-out or order-out generation?" I questioned.

"No, it has to enchant all generations. It should rekindle their fountain of youth and memories; make them young-at-heart again; and stimulate their enthusiasm and passion."

"That reminds me of Dr. Charles Jarvis, who said that he tells his wife every morning how beautiful she looks. It is hard to pretend in life that everything is beautiful time and again, by doing the same routine people have been doing for the past 10, 20, or 30 years for Valentine's Day and expect to have a sparkling new experience."

"Yeah! That is called insanity. We want to help people rejuvenate their passion that they had when they met for the first time," she insisted.

"I have a perfect Valentine's Day plan for your listeners. Let us set the scene. Take your jacket, let's go!"

"Where?" she asked.

"To create an experience they can celebrate for years to come,"

I said.

"Where are we going?"

"First stop, the grocery store."

"For what?" she asked.

"To get some romantic ingredients."

"Are you serious? I thought you were going to recommend some fine diner."

"Well, we are going to give them the best dining experience. It is called dine-in in the comfort of your own home!"

"Are you sure?"

"Sonia, believe me. They are going to get a firsthand experience at doing things for each other, rather than ordering stuff."

"I don't know where you are going with this!" she said doubtfully.

"First, let's stop at the fresh fruits and vegetable section."

"And then?"

"We can pick up romaine lettuce, spinach leaves, dark red and yellow bell peppers, onions, tomatoes, cucumbers, cantaloupes, and mangoes."

"What is that for?" She looked surprised.

"Do you need an answer for everything?"

"I thought you said that they should do things together. If so, both need to know what the other person is thinking."

"Well, you got me there. The lettuce is rich in fiber. The dark pigmented bell peppers are rich in antioxidants, cantaloupe has anti-aging ingredients. These agents are supposed to help rejuvenate their youth."

"With just one serving?" She laughed.

"No, but this is a new beginning. That is why they are going to have a Perfect Valentine Day Treat. Next, let's pick up some olive oil and walnuts."

"Are you nuts?" she asked.

"You see, olive oil is the best cooking oil, with its rich monounsaturated fatty acids that keep cholesterol down."

"What about walnuts?"

"Walnuts are rich in omega-3 fatty acids, which lower cholesterol. Besides, roasted walnuts taste great with a fancy salad."

"Who is going to make the salad?" she asked.

"The couple!" I said. "We need some French or Italian red wine."

"Why not beer or whisky?" Sonia quizzed.

"No, they do not give the same sensual experience as a glass of white or red wine on a romantic evening. Besides, red wine has been shown to reduce the incidence of heart disease in the French population."

"Are we talking about a Valentine's Day treat or a lecture on healthy foods?"

"Well, I am showing you how to find the beauty in the beast," I said.

"As long as you see it, let us continue!" Sarcastically, she laughed.

"Trust me, if you follow this dialogue to the end, you will know what I am talking about."

"Next, please?" She could not wait.

"Shall we move to the meat section and pick up some protein?"

"Could you please speak English?"

"Do you want chicken, lean beef, lamb, or fish?"

"Nik, since you have an answer for everything, why don't you help me choose."

"I do not have the answer to everything. I question everything just like you do. The plan is for them to grill the meat for the main course of the dinner. Therefore, we need to select a lean-cut meat so we can enjoy their Valentine's Day dinner. Chicken has less fat than beef, and so does lean lamb. In fact, fish such as salmon, tuna, or mackerel have high omega-3 fatty acid levels, which help lower cholesterol. I think you should be fine with any one of those choices. You also need your favorite spices to marinate the meat before grilling it."

"Then?" She did not look like someone who wanted to stand in front of a grill.

"We could also pick up some carrots, which are rich in vitamins. Let's select some beans that can be steam cooked to perfection to go with the main course."

"How do you know about all these cooking tips?" She looked curious.

"I watch many cooking channels. However, I do not recommend the amount of fat and butter they use."

"What about the dessert?" she said, with a broad smile on her face.

"Yeah! What is a Valentine's Day dinner without some divine chocolate dessert? Let's pick up some ice cream, chocolate chips and chocolate syrup."

"Did you say you are a heart doctor?" she quipped.

"We'll talk about it later. Now, let's head home and transform the kitchen and the living room into a romantic get-away or hide-away."

"How are we going to do that?" she questioned.

"First, drop off the kids at your sister's."

"My sister is not a baby-sitter."

"Well, if the price is right?" I joked.

"I get the message."

"Next, the couple will take part in preparing the romantic appetizer, the main entrée, and the dessert."

"Nik, that is too much work. No one is going to fall for that!"

"That is how their romantic relationship started. Doing something special for each other. It is time to relive those moments."

"What do they do next?" She pretended innocence.

"Decorate the dining table with a nice tablecloth, light up a couple of candles that emit a romantic aroma, and turn the lights down. One person will pour the red wine into the glasses, while the other person turns on soft, soothing music. Now, they cut a few slices of cheese, celery, cucumber, and carrots for appetizer."

"That sounds interesting." She began to show some curiosity.

"While one person marinates the meat, the other person will prepare the salad with lettuce, cucumbers, olives, cheese, roasted walnuts, olive oil, and fresh peppers."

"That should make people think about the last time they treated each other to that special occasion. Now, you are right. Anybody can order out a dinner," she said.

"Next, they will steam-cook the vegetables and mix them with onions, salt and pepper sautéed in olive oil."

"What about the main course?" She couldn't wait.

"It's coming. They will put the marinated meat, be it chicken, lamb chops, sirloin, or salmon, on the grill and turn on the timer. Meantime, they continue to enjoy their wine and cheese as the evening turns more passionate."

"What about the cell phones?" she laughed, looking at her text messages.

"Just silence them. Better yet, hide them in the closet. The only thing they may be able to feel or hear will be their own heartbeats, in sync with the soft, soothing music in the background, while their eyes gaze at the beautiful dark blue sky lit with a full moon. When the grill timer goes off, they turn the meat over and let it cook for the desired time on the other side," I said.

"Now, let me guess, they get their salad and dinner plates ready on the dinner table that is illuminated by the candles radiating the romantic aroma. But, Nik, did we forget the carbs? I see no carbohydrates."

"Are you kidding? Everyone wants to look his or her best on Valentine's Day. They do not want to look or feel bloated. That is why we have put the carbs on hold for this special evening," I said.

"Nik, while they are having their delightful dinner, they need to have a topic to engage both of them and bring them closer," Sonia said.

"I think they can talk about their next vacation spot they want to visit, or the fun stuff they wanted to do together," I said.

"That sounds more personal and intimate. I am sure the delicious salad and the sizzling grilled meat should serve as the fuel for such a conversation," Sonia said.

"Once they finish their delectable dinner, as usual, the man will attend to the dishes, while the lady scoops out ice cream into one large glass bowl, adds cubes of cantaloupes, sliced strawberries, green raisins, and of course bits of roasted walnuts. Then the most important ingredient of all for Valentine's Day, the hot melted dark chocolate will drape the surface," I said.

"As they delicately dip their spoons into the dessert bowl, their memories will freeze the moment in time. Then, as they put the spoons filled with chocolate ice cream into each other's mouths, again their vivid souls will seize the moment of Valentine's Day Zen," she said.

"It should expose their sublime adoration for each other. You may also notice that their intense eyes will be doing all the talking, while their lips are sealed with the hot melting chocolate," I said.

"How do you know?" she asked.

"Just imagination. It does not cost anything. But it will leave an eternal memory in the sands of time. By the way, Sonia, you are doing so good when it comes to the romantic part, I should have let you lead this dialog from the beginning," I said.

"Nik, that hot melting chocolate should energize them to go to a park, take a wild walk, throw snow or mudballs at each other, and reenact their first passionate interlude."

"Sonia, I could not have said it better."

"Thanks, Nik. Tomorrow is Valentine's Day. And I am late for my grocery shopping." Having said that, Sonia drove off in her BMW, into the sunset.

Afterthoughts: Why not extend that experience to every evening? Dinner is more than just another meal. It is the final reward for your existence and effort. It is an experience you look forward to while working all day long.

When we talk about a fine dining experience, we generally say, "We had a wonderful time," "It was a beautiful evening," or "It was awesome," instead of saying, "The dessert was very, very, very sweet," or "The meat was well-cooked." It is the total experience that counts and makes the difference. Your home banquet should be special, and should appeal to all your five senses plus a sense of humor. It should be your mission to create an everyday experience better than that of a five-star restaurant at your own *Dining-inn,* using your kitchen and breakfast room.

You are the movie director and it is up to you to create an ambience that matches a steak house, a seafood place, an ethnic restaurant, the beach, or at sea on a love boat. Since the choices are limited only by your imagination, be bold and daring. Do something different that will be more rewarding and fulfilling than just driving across town to grab an unhealthy piece of meat.

A Heart Healthy Lifestyle may mean changing your culture, if not your religion, when it comes to reprogramming your habits and appetites, as well as restocking your kitchen, refrigerator, and pantry.

Of course, you may have to take up multiple roles, such as an intelligent shopper, an interior decorator, a chef, a waiter, a host, and a guest. I recognize it is a lot to expect from you at the end of a long day. Still, the pleasant voyage taken with your dinner partner is worth every minute of your effort. This grants you an opportunity to spend quality time with your partner, while you two become the architects of your own heart healthy dining delight. Before you can reach that zenith, though, you must invest some time, effort, and money to transform your kitchen and dining room into a dream world.

If you do not own a convection oven, invest in a modern countertop UltraVection oven that grills food quickly and crisply. Grilling aids in preparing heart healthy meals, while reducing cooking and cleaning time.

Marinate your lean-cut chicken breast, trimmed fillet mignon, lamb or pork chops, or fish overnight. Be liberal with your spices and go light on the oil, since meat already contains hidden fat. Cook the meat in the oven for 6 to10 minutes on each side.

Steam-cook your vegetables on a stove or in a microwave oven. Season your vegetables with a touch of olive oil or Benecol (a heart healthy margarine substitute containing a plant stanol) along with salt, pepper, and your favorite spices.

As you can see, I have spent a substantial amount of time discussing the dinner aesthetics, instead of dwelling on the quantity or richness of food itself in terms of butter, cholesterol, or sugar. This is what I call a life-rejuvenation revolution, replacing those old and unhealthy lifestyles that previously had clogged your consciousness.

After dinner, you can turn up the music and have a relaxing, romantic after-dinner dance with your partner, burning those carb calories while loosening up your muscles and joints. Watch out! This experience could be addictive. However, it is better to be addicted to a heart healthy habit than to be enslaved to old routines. Or, you could wind down your evening in the company of your spouse, on the couch. That is far better than driving back from a distant restaurant in a disgusted, lonely mood, because your spouse is still fuming at you for not paying the gas bill on time last month or for hitting on the waitress.

One day, when you invite your family and friends over for an evening, they will be astonished at your creativity, and admire your aesthetic taste all evening. Your tranquil environment and pleasant company will leave many fond memories. This could be an opportune occasion to share with them the amazing Heart Healthy Lifestyle you learned from Dr. Nik's book, and what a difference it has made in your life. Don't forget to apply your new lifestyle even when you are eating out.

Why is dining at your own inn so essential, you may ask? If you are married and both of you work, opportunities for dining at your inn are rare. You may have dinner meetings twice a week with your business group, while your spouse has her lady's night out every Wednesday. Then you have to take part in the kids' football games — top that off with three weekend parties. That leaves you with maybe one or two days a week to enjoy a heart healthy, home-cooked meal. I bet you will be very sorry if you spoil that chance.

Dining in at your own inn has several advantages:

- For one, you don't have to drive halfway across the city.
- You don't need to wait in line for an hour and a half because you are number 93.
- You don't have to share your lungs with the smokers.
- You don't have to wait outside in the freezing cold.
- You won't have to face an entourage of restaurant models: check-in girl, water girl, menu boy, and finally the real fellow who is actually supposed to serve you.
- You can save on gas expenses.
- You save time.

- There won't be any interruptions by the staff.
- You don't have to stuff yourself to justify the price and the drive.
- You will know who cooked your food.
- Your food is less likely to be under or overcooked, burned, or raw.
- The food will be warm and ready when you want it.
- You don't have to attract the waitress to pay attention to your needs.
- You can avoid a noisy and crowded place.

You get the picture.

Dining-Out Choices

Here are some heart healthy choices to consider when preparing your multi-course dinner at your inn.

Appetizers: Make sure your appetizers are light and simple. You can munch on an ounce of nuts, which provides you with protein and polyunsaturated fats. One ounce of nuts has 12 to 14 grams of fat. Macadamia nuts are high in fats and should be avoided. You also can nibble on vegetables such as tomatoes, cucumbers, or cauliflower seasoned with salt and pepper or dipped in your favorite low-fat dressing. Make your conversation the main appetizing ingredient for the happy hour. Let your tongue do more talking and less chewing. As a matter of fact, the purpose of the happy hour is to socialize with other people, not so much with food. You could always stuff yourself equally well at home, on the road, or in the back seat of a car. But, you cannot talk or shake hands with your friends if you attach yourself to the edge of the cocktail table and embark on an appetite indulgence expedition.

Avoid isolating yourself from the rest of the group and complaining that no one talks to you and this world is a miserable place. There is no such thing as a miserable world. The world is exactly as you see and feel it. It is up to you to make your own world. If you make a wonderful and joyful world around you, people will come spend time with you and have fun.

Drinks: As mentioned elsewhere, red wine has been shown to reduce heart disease risk because of its antioxidant properties. However, white wine does not provide the same benefits. Anyway, a glass of red or white wine (considering that you are old enough to drink) should add some pizzazz to your dining experience. By all means, drink plenty of water before, during, and after the dinner. You may enjoy a hot cup of freshly brewed coffee or tea, if that makes you happy. Avoid soft drinks loaded with empty calories.

Appetizers
Dry roasted soy nuts (1 oz.)
Peanuts or almonds (1/2 to 1 oz.)
Celery
Cucumber (one)
Berries
Apple (1), or other fruits (1 or 2)
Plums
Dry-roasted chickpeas (1/2 cup)
Spicy tofu cubes
Pumpkin seeds (1 oz.)
Vegetables with low-fat vegetable dips

Main items
(Skinless, lean, fat-trimmed, and boneless)
Grilled salmon, mackerel, or tuna (4 oz.)
Fajita chicken with whole-wheat tortillas
Fajita beef with whole-wheat tortillas
Sirloin steak (4 oz., roasted with your favorite spices)
Grilled lean beef (4 oz.)
Grilled chicken breast (seasoned with lemon pepper, 4 oz.)
Lean grilled meat or trimmed pork chops (4 oz.)
Grilled lean lamb chops (4 oz.)
Shish kabobs (beef, chicken, or lamb)
Roasted lean lamb or beef (4 oz.)
Roasted skinless chicken (4 oz.)
Grilled shrimp (6-8 pieces)

Ground beef (2% fat)
Ground turkey (2 to 7% fat)
Veggie burgers

Beans
All types of beans (½ cup)
Lima beans (½ cup)
Chickpeas (½ cup)
Kidney beans (½ cup)
Black-eyed peas (½ cup)
Soybean hamburger patties

Carbs
Basmati rice (½ cup)
Pasta (½ cup)
Bread (1 to 2 slices)
High fiber tortillas (10 g fiber per tortilla)

Vegetables
Spinach (1 cup)
Asparagus
String beans
Cauliflower
Broccoli
Okra (½ cup)
Mixed vegetables
Eggplant

Fruits
(please, be sure to add the fruit calories to your total carb count)
Pear
Apple
Banana
Mango
Strawberries
Cantaloupe

Drinks
Wine (6 to 8 oz.)
Lemon-juice with a sugar substitute
Iced tea with a sweetener
Water
Coffee or tea
Rum-flavored diet Coke! How about that?

Side dishes
Steamed vegetables, fruits, and nuts
Cottage cheese (fat-free) in place of potatoes
A low-calorie whole-wheat bread
Green salad
Sugar-free Jell-O salads

Desserts
Fruit plate
Pear slices (½ cup)
Gelatin desserts with sweetener
Homemade desserts (using a sweetener and Benecol)
Low-fat ice cream
Low-fat yogurt, sherbet, or puddings

Salads & Soups
Dinner salad
Greek salad with light dressing
Caesar's salad with light dressing or lime-pepper
Salsa
Soups: lentil, pea, onion, bean, beef, or vegetable
   (Soups have high salt content. Avoid them if you have blood
   pressure problems.)

Salad dressings
Olive oil (1 tsp.)
Light dressing (20 calories) in place of regular dressing (170

calories)

Spices
Lime-pepper
Red chili powder
Seasoning: Cajun, Greek, Italian, tandoori, etc.

Shopping List

Music: Gather the most romantic, soothing, and relaxing music compilation from around the world from your local music store. Copy the songs onto an MP3 player. Then, with a touch of a button, you can have your cherished tranquil music filling your heart and mind for hours and hours without interruption. Select the random option so the sequence of songs is never the same each day.

Table setup: Make your dinner table as aesthetic and attractive as any dining table you have seen in the finest restaurants. Invest in a fine set of silverware with sharp steak knives. They will last for a decade. One spouse may be on business trips thirteen months a year, while the other spouse has to attend business meetings five nights a week. Therefore, planning for that one special night is essential to gather long-lasting memories.

Lighting: Replace those blinding two-hundred-watt light bulbs with soft, colorful sixty-watt light bulbs. It is a good time to invest in a stylish chandelier that matches the new décor of your dining table. Color coordination is very important. Men are born color-clueless according to some ladies, if you have not noticed. To avoid making numerous trips to the store in vain, consult with your lady before you invest in a gold chandelier that doesn't match your bronze décor. If both of you visit the store at the same time, then let your lady do the talking and shopping while you do the paying. It is better to settle your differences in front of the store manager in a civilized style— according to the lady's rule—that is less stressful on your heart and nerves. It is part of heart healthy living — compromise, on your part. What part don't you understand? While you are at the store, purchase a dimmer switch so that the illumination in your dining room can be tuned in sync with your romantic vibrations for that day.

Serving utensils: Make sure that your daily serving utensils are of a good, durable quality with a shimmering shine. If you don't go out to eat for at least three months, you will save enough money to invest in a brand-new silver serving set. Use wine glasses for water as well as for wine, like the five-star restaurants do. This adds a whole new dimension to your dining experience. Remember, it is the ambiance and the total experience that we are trying to emphasize; an evening should be much more than just biting each other's head of before the night falls.

Plan for the week: When you serve yourself a sizzling-hot, made-to-order, best gourmet dinner at your own dining table, your sensation is sure to climax. In order to realize this sensual dream, visit your local grocery store or health food store with your spouse to select lean-cut meats suitable for grilling or baking. Marinate the meat and put each day's quota in a Ziploc freezer bag. Then, just transfer the meat that you are planning to eat the next day to the refrigerator so the meat is defrosted and well marinated by the time you are ready to grill. Do not leave the meat outside at room temperature, as it is likely to get spoiled by the time you return home. You could also season your frozen vegetables and move them to the refrigerator the previous night. They will be ready for steam-cooking and seasoning in the evening.

Cooking lessons: Watch various cooking channels to learn hundreds of different ways to grill your favorite foods instead of frying them in a floating grease pond. Set aside a Sunday to search Google under the heading "grilling." Learn how different ethnic groups marinate their meats using exotic spices in a thousand different ways to accent their distinctive ethnic flavor, using a trouble-free grilling process. Thus, you can enjoy foods from all around the world in your own kitchen. Turn your kitchen into an international cooking laboratory specializing in dinner cuisine from around the world, where the process of cooking a variety of foods takes center stage above overindulgence in unhealthy foods. If you would like to know how to make chicken rice the Indian way, log onto YouTube and type, "Indian chicken rice." The chef will give you a full demonstration on how to make chicken rice.

Food and TV: Eating in front of a television is the greatest threat to your beltline or hip perimeter. People are generally addicted to both television and food. However, when you combine these two addictions, you are likely to lose control over both. In other words, you cannot stop until the game is over or the house is free of edibles. Then, you will start searching for the snacks, nuts, or anything else that you can get your hands on. In desperate situations, I have seen people chewing on aluminum foil to get through the game so that they can go out after the game for a festive food-stuffing ceremony! Oh! Did I mention alcohol?

Never eat food when you are angry: That is a dangerous approach to settle your score, since your appetite and calorie count will always lose in the end. A better alternative is to take a walk away from the kitchen for a couple of hours or a cold shower until the tap runs dry or your skin turns blue. Lowering your temper by thirty to forty degrees is critical before you move back into the kitchen. Law enforcement people hate to walk over broken china or half-baked potatoes. If you have not realized that, only you will have to clean up the mess before the boss arrives for an inspection! Calmly analyze the situation that ignited the passionate anger and how much you were responsible for that. Then take appropriate steps so you never fuel such a situation from your side. An opponent without opposition soon loses steam. Automatically, you win!

Overstuffing: Make sure that you do not overstuff yourself late at night. Excess fat stays longer in the stomach and produces acid reflex into the esophagus, causing heartburn in the middle of the night. Over time, the acid may cause erosion of the esophagus, leading to esophagitis, which is hard to control. Finish your dinner at least a couple of hours before you retire to bed and walk as much as possible; better yet, take a nice walk around the neighborhood after dinner (provided your neighborhood is not infested with strange rocks; you get the picture). Walking helps you to burn the extra calories, exercises your muscles, and helps you to get a good night's sleep. Finishing your dinner early gives you more time to be proactive in how you use the rest of the evening. You can use this time to plan your next day or next several days. Write down all the things that you have on your mind before you go to sleep. That will allow your unconscious mind to work on it while you enjoy a good night's sleep.

Slim meals: Some of the points regarding low-calorie diets have been covered else where. Here we have added a few more features to emphasize that not all low-calorie foods are equal. Beware of the content of low-calorie meals. Most of them stress low-fat, which means they are loaded with a disproportionate amount of carbohydrates. Do not be misled by low-fat or fat-free claims. You need to pay special attention to carbohydrates, salt, and cholesterol. Most frozen foods have a much higher salt content compared to their fresh counterparts. The sauce and creams are usually made of carbohydrate, and they add a lot of empty calories. As a rule of thumb, if a Lean Cuisine has more than 30 grams of carbohydrates, then look for frozen lunchmeat such as fatless chicken, beef, or turkey. Then add your own vegetables so you become an educated consumer rather than falling prey to those marketing catch phrases such as low-fat and fat-free. If the package reads 60 to 80 grams of carbohydrates, then don't touch it. Move to the next item. I realize a landscape worker pushing a lawn mover for 8 to 10 hours a day in the heat, will need a lot of calories. Believe me, he will not be shopping in the Lean Cuisine section.

Grilling class: Though traditionally, outdoor grilling has been a man's pride, indoor grilling is a completely different dimension for a man. You will certainly need the assistance of your spouse for indoor grilling. Most men know how to operate an outside grill, but they are like a fish out of water when they are exposed to indoor grills. Without indoor grilling talents, a man can easily convert a prime rib into a charcoal cube in the absence of his spouse's assistance and guidance. In an indoor cooking situation, there is a tendency for a man to lose track of time because it is not mission-critical when cooking outdoors. His mental calculations may be so far off base, he may not realize that he has been "cooking" for an hour with no food on the kitchen grill.

Joint cooking: Preparing dinner together also allows for lovely grill side conversations. For a man who has had no domestic training in the kitchen and is now forced into position as a chef, I will mention a few helpful hints that I have learned over the years. When cooking anywhere, outside or inside, leave the meat simmering on low heat for the last few minutes to give the juices time to "settle in" and to preserve the meat's moisture and tenderness. Also, it might be a culture shock for you to cook in a smoke-free environment. At first, you might have a little trouble thinking outside of the haze you are used to with backyard grilling. However, get used to it. When grilling outdoors, you might have to fight charcoal smoke or cigarette smoke, but indoor grilling will overcome both the charcoal smoke and certainly the cigarette smoke—another step toward your Heart Healthy Lifestyle!

While the meat is being cooked, don't stick your finger into the oven to taste the chicken breast, like you normally would do in an outdoor setting. Your spouse will direct you when and how to taste the food cooking on the time-regulated, indoor grill. Some dining etiquette is in order here.

When you are officially instructed to inspect the food, make sure to use a spoon or a fork and let the food cool before you burn your taste buds. Be very gentle with your comments or suggestions, lest you wreck the rest of the evening.

Chapter 12

Heart Structure & Engineering
Engineering marvels of heart structure

The good Almighty created the human heart first. In the process, he gathered so much information, he decided to create all the branches of engineering that we have today. Yet, what engineers create today cannot even come close to the Almighty's marvel.

The fetal heart develops from a tiny tube in the mother's womb at 12 weeks into gestation into a miniature 4-cylinder pump that beats, beat after beat, for the rest of life. Can you think of anything that engineering has created that can match this endurance, tenacity, and reliability? Even a space shuttle, the greatest engineering marvel, does not even come close to what a heart muscle the size of a fist can accomplish for more than a century in some patients. Let us look at some of the engineering concepts that have evolved from the heart's function.

Mechanical engineering and the human heart: Imagine attaching a mechanical pump to the end of a flexible tube. With the energy generated by the pump, you are able to move fluid from point A to point B. The amount of fluid moved is based on the energy produced by the pump and the resistance offered by the flexible tube. In this "heart," the amount of fluid equates to the blood pumped with each heartbeat. The tube represents the blood vessels, and the flexibility represents the vascular (blood vessel) resistance. So, the vascular resistance is measured indirectly by the simple blood pressure machine. The vascular resistance forms the basis of high blood pressure. So, getting back to your engineering concept, if you want to reduce high blood pressure, you can do so by reducing vascular resistance or the force with which the heart pumps. The beta-blocker drugs reduce the force by which the heart pumps, while water pills and ACE inhibitors work by reducing the vascular resistance.

Electrical engineering and the human heart: To light up a city, we need power plants, thousands of miles of an electrical grid, relay stations, transformers, and generators. The human heart, about the size of your fist, contains all these elements within itself, from a generator, a transmitter, and an electrical grid to a relay station. The heart generates its own electrical impulse by specialized heart muscle cells located in strategic locations, the most important of which is the sinus node. It is located at the junction of the right upper chamber and the main vein coming from the head and neck (superior vena cava), and generates the impulse that initiates the electrical activity of the heart that leads to muscle contraction, which is the mechanical end result. The impulse travels through a network of specialized muscle fibers (the "electrical grid") to the relay station, called the AV node. The AV node acts as a delay station to hold the impulse until the mechanical function of the upper chambers is completed. After the upper chambers pump the blood into the lower chambers, the electrical impulse activates the lower chambers.

Civil engineering and the human heart: The civil engineering involves architectural, structural, mechanical, electrical and plumbing components. The heart structure is another example of an engineering marvel in the architectural and structural engineering fields. There is nothing that parallels the architecture of the heart, where all four chambers (cylinders) are glued together. The heart muscle is designed in such a manner that when the upper chambers squeeze simultaneously, the lower chambers relax. When the lower chambers squeeze, the upper chambers relax. It is based on hydraulic principle, when one set of chambers squeezes, the other set relaxes to accommodate the influx of blood and vice versa. When the heart muscle gets weak due to a heart attack or high blood pressure, the heart loses its pumping efficiency, leading to heart failure.

We talked about the electrical system in the heart. Now, let us focus our attention on the plumbing system in the heart. The heart itself acts as the pump to the entire plumbing system in the body. The arteries carry the pure blood, oxygen, and nutrients to the rest of the body. The veins return the impure blood to the heart, which pumps it to the lungs to re-oxygenate the blood and remove waste products such as carbon dioxide.

Most of us have experienced clogged plumbing at one time or another. And, I also have seen arteries of people in their seventies that are clean as a whistle. How could that be possible, given the fact the plumbing system in the body is most convoluted with twists and turns? No man-made lubricating system comes close to the efficiency of the plumbing system in the body. Blood, with its ability to stay liquid and not stick to the blood vessels, yet allow nutrients to move in and out of the blood vessels, is truly amazing. Yet we, with all our habits such as unhealthy diet, smoking, and lack of exercise, ruin these blood vessels, leading to heart attacks, strokes, kidney failure or peripheral artery disease. The inner lining of the heart chambers prevents the blood from clotting, even though the blood is subjected to such high pressure during squeezing. The heart and the veins have valves that allow blood to flow in only one direction so that the blood moves in the forward direction with each heartbeat.

Computer engineering and the human heart: Microsoft, Sun, Cisco, and Google pale in significance compared with the hardware and software engineering that has gone to heart function. The heart is hardwired to the brain, so that they can communicate with each other instantaneously, in real time. The heart and the brain have true intelligence (not artificial), by which they can incorporate past experiences into future actions and reactions. The heart is programmed to respond to every conceivable challenge, even before we face them, and is fully engraved into the system even before a baby is born. The heart knows when to slow down, when to speed up, and even when to stop. The beauty of the system is that with training, the unwanted reactions can be tamed. With exercise, we can train our heart to respond with a slower heart rate response. Similarly, with training and confidence, we can reduce our palpitations during stressful situations. The software programming is continuously upgrading itself with each experience so that you do not have to buy an upgrade every year.

Chemical engineering and the human heart: The human body is the greatest chemical factory in the world and the heart is in the center of it. Most of the heart function is dependent on chemical messengers that are controlled and released by the endocrine glands. When you want to run, the brain sends signals to the adrenal glands to produce more adrenaline, which stimulates the sinus node to speed up the heart rate. At the same time, it dilates the blood vessels to accommodate more blood supply to the working muscles. On the other hand, when we are sleeping, the body sends a signal to slow the heart rate as the demand is reduced, to conserve energy.

When we start a car, the engine uses oil, which is converted into energy to move the pistons. Interestingly enough, the heart muscle also uses fatty acids (oil) for its continuous energy needs. When there is increased demand, the heart uses glucose for immediate energy needs. So, the heart has been using a dual source of energy for thousands of years. This is the basis on which the concepts of new hybrid cars were conceived.

Friction is an inherent problem with many moving parts and accounts for wear and tear. Not so when it comes to the heart. You could be jogging at 6 miles per hour, with your heart beating at 150 beats per minute against your chest wall, and yet it does not suffer any trauma. It is surrounded by a pericardial sack (a thin sheath that covers the heart) with a thin layer of fluid, which acts as a shock absorber so that the heart simply glides with each beat with very little friction. Now you know where engineering came from!

Chapter 13

Chest Pain Causes
Is it a heart attack?

Common Causes of Chest Pain

During the past 25 years of practice in cardiology, I have come across people with chest pain ranging in age from 12 to over 100. The causes and the management vary greatly based on age, sex, underlying physical or emotional factors, and family history, among many other factors.

School children: We get calls to see schoolchildren as young as 12 years old who experience chest pain, especially with exertion. Most of us have heard about young athletes dying on the basketball courts. Most of the time, the chest pain may not be related to any real heart disease. The child may be out of shape or may be exerting beyond capacity, which can cause chest pain in most people. It is not uncommon for children after a bout of cold, congestion and persistent cough to experience chest pain from sore ribs or muscles. Most of the time, the chest pain is harmless and self limiting. If the pain persists, consult with your physician. If your physician detects any abnormalities in the rhythm, heart sounds, or murmurs, then consult with a pediatric cardiologist; a 2D echocardiogram can be helpful in excluding any significant heart disease.

Young adults: Young adults between the ages of 20 and 35 also may have chest pains because of various causes. Let us take a look at some common problems that we have seen in our daily practice.

Pleurisy: Occasionally, people can develop pleurisy or inflammation of the lining that covers the lungs, which can cause pain made worse by deep breathing. It occurs in association with a viral syndrome and lasts for a few days. It responds very well to anti-inflammatory agents such as Motrin or Indocin.

Pericarditis: A similar inflammatory process can involve the pericardium, the tissue that covers the heart muscle, resulting in pericarditis, which can cause chest pain. The pericarditis pain intensifies with deep breathing and is associated with characteristic EKG changes.

Hypertrophic cardiomyopathy: This is a rare condition with increased thickness of the left ventricular wall and the septum that separates the right and the left ventricles. It causes chest pain on exertion, shortness of breath, irregular heart rhythms, and rarely, sudden death. An EKG may show increased voltage due to the thick heart muscle. A 2D echocardiogram study can enable us to diagnose the presence of hypertrophic cardiomyopathy. Students engaging in vigorous activities such as basketball, football, or other athletics, would definitely benefit from a 2D echocardiogram, especially if the person has experienced chest pain.

Syndrome X: Some young ladies in their thirties and forties may experience chest pain. A complete cardiovascular examination including a stress test and cardiac catheterization (putting catheters in the heart, to image the heart and blood vessels) may fail to reveal significant coronary artery disease. These women have an increased risk of future cardiovascular events, and they must be treated aggressively as though they had a heart problem and encouraged to lose weight, if they are overweight. They should also be treated with medicines for blood pressure and cholesterol, and encouraged to exercise.

Conditions mimicking chest pain from heart disease: Several conditions also can cause chest pain that can mimic heart disease. However, it is impossible, based on the history alone, to differentiate chest pain arising from other causes from those arising from a real heart problem. Careful examination, EKG, 2D echocardiogram and a stress test can help us differentiate the conditions.

Acid reflux: It is a common problem that can lead to heartburn, which can mimic heart pains. Most people would seek comfort, thinking the pain is because of acid reflux, and get used to routine antacid use. If you are having any discomfort in your chest, it is advisable to get a complete cardiovascular evaluation including a stress test. Long-term use of antacids is not a solution even if you are having acid reflux. Consult with a gastroenterologist if you have symptoms for more than 6 to 8 weeks despite being treated with antacids.

Gallstone symptoms: Gall bladder symptoms can mimic coronary artery disease symptoms. We have seen people admitted to the hospital with what appeared to be a gallbladder attack in a person as young as in the thirties to realize that it was actually a heart attack. Getting an electrocardiogram in all patients would help to rule out any significant acute cardiac events.

Anxiety: Anxiety can mimic just about any heart disease symptom, or for that matter, any type of symptom. We have seen people experience chest pains when one of the family members is diagnosed to have heart disease or suffer from a heart attack. It is normal to feel chest pain during a period of anxiety and the anxiety itself makes the symptoms worse. The more you worry about it, the more intense the symptoms become. After thorough cardiovascular evaluation, if there is no evidence for a serious heart disease, your physician may prescribe a short course of tranquilizers to help you get over the acute anxiety situation.

Mitral Valve Prolapse

Some time ago, a 26-year-old college student by the name Sandy came to my office with chest pain after she had a breakup with her boyfriend. I said, "Hi, Sandy, how are you?"

"Not so good," she said.

"What brings you here?"

"Lately, I've been having chest pain. It's located on the left side. It comes and goes. I also feel fluttering in the chest. Sometimes, I feel dizzy." She sounded anxious.

"How long did you have these symptoms?" I said.

"I had them for the past several months. They weren't that severe. Now, they're coming on every day. My sister had the same symptoms. She was told that she had a floppy valve. I have no idea what it means!" she said.

"What brings on these symptoms?" I said.

"Stress. Like when I'm studying for finals, or when I fight with my sister," she said.

"Anything else?" I leaned forward.

"Yes, I feel weak, tired all the time, and restless at times."

"Any other type of stress?" I said.

"I just broke up with my boyfriend, if you consider that as stress." She smiled.

"Oh! Yeah, that can give chest pain to both of you," I said.

"What is this floppy valve I hear about? Do you think I might have the same problem?" She looked worried.

Listening to her heart, I said, "I hear a click."

"What is a click?" she said.

"It is an extra sound produced by the mitral valve."

"Do you hear anything else?"

"I hear some extra beats."

"What does all that mean in English?" she said.

"You most likely have mitral valve prolapse," I continued.

"What is mitral valve prolapse?" She could not wait for the answer.

"In this condition, the mitral leaflets are loose and floppy," I said.

"Is it the same thing as what my sister has?" she asked.

"Yes. Sometimes, we see them with several family members. Normally, the mitral valve closes in a straight line. However, in mitral valve prolapse, the leaflets are loose and lax and they bulge into the left upper chamber, causing the click," I said.

"How do people get this condition?" She asked.

"It is a form of a congenital abnormality. People with connective tissue disorder or Marfan's syndrome are at an increased risk of developing mitral valve prolapse. Patients develop symptoms in their twenties and thirties. It is a common condition occurring in two to three percent of adults."

"How do you confirm your diagnosis?" She looked suspicious.

"Well, let's go to the next room and perform an echocardiogram of the heart."

While performing the echocardiogram, I pointed out, "See that mitral valve that looks like a sail opening and closing?"

"That's amazing. That is my heart? And, that's the mitral valve?" she said, gazing at the ultrasound monitor.

"Yes, you see your mitral valve bulging into the left upper chamber with each heartbeat?" I asked.

"It looks like a parachute!" she said.

"You should have gone into medicine! That is exactly how we describe it," I said.

"Is this dangerous?" she asked.

"Generally not. Rarely, the valve may begin to leak, causing a heart murmur," I said.

"Then what happens?"

"In one or two percent of people, the valve leak may get worse to the point where it may have to be replaced." I paused.

"You're a big help. How do you treat this condition?" she asked.

"Find a new boyfriend!" I raised my eyebrows.

"Besides that?" she made a grim face.

"No, really, the symptoms come and go. Sometimes they are exacerbated during periods of stress. Some patients may have no symptoms at all. It can be treated with a simple beta-blocker such as Atenolol or Lopressor," I said.

"What is that? How does it work and how long do I have to take it?" She had a look of aversion.

"The beta-blocker slows the heart rate, reduces the strain on the heart muscle and relieves the chest pain. You have to stay on the pills long-term. When people stop the pills, the symptoms may come back. Some people stop the pills and don't have symptoms for a long time. Beta-blockers are very benign and cause no harm," I said.

"How do you fix the valve?"

"We cannot fix the valve. We can only control the symptoms."

"Then, how do you prevent the valve from getting worse?"

"That is a good question. I still think you should have gone into medicine. There is nothing to prevent the valve from getting worse. Fortunately, only one or two percent of people with MVP develop a severe leak that may need surgery," I tried to reassure her.

"That's it, finished?" She looked surprised.

"One more thing, people who have mitral valve prolapse with moderate leak or regurgitation may be advised antibiotics before they have dental work or surgery," I said.

"I'm glad that you mentioned this. My sister wanted me to ask you why we need antibiotics before any dental work," she said.

"Since the valve is loose and lax, it is more prone to trauma. When you have dental work or surgery, there is a release of bacteria into the bloodstream that can infect the valve. However, the American Heart Association does not recommend routine antibiotic prophylaxis for garden-variety mitral valve prolapse," I said, "based on the 2007 recommendations."

"That makes sense." She smiled.

"Here is the prescription for Atenolol 25 mg one daily by mouth," I said.

"Do I still have to take this pill? My chest pain is gone."

"You may want to keep the pills handy, just in case your symptoms come back, or your old boyfriend wants to come back in your life."

"You need help!" she said as she walked to the checkout counter.

Chapter 14

Cholesterol & Triglycerides

Classification of Cholesterol

Cholesterol performs vital functions in the body, serving as a building block for many important hormones such as estrogen and testosterone, as well as natural steroids. Cholesterol is an important component of cells and the oil glands that protect the skin from drying. It helps provide structure for the cell membrane. High cholesterol is the number one risk factor for heart disease.

Cholesterol comes from two main sources: our diet and our liver. The dietary cholesterol comes from eggs and meat products. The liver produces cholesterol from raw materials in the blood. Saturated fats tend to raise LDL cholesterol levels. Liver is the main organ where cholesterol is produced. When high glycemic index carbohydrates and saturated fats are consumed, they are broken down into smaller components that are used by the liver to produce cholesterol. However, the body makes enough cholesterol, so dietary cholesterol is not essential.

Until the cholesterol is needed, it circulates in the blood. Cholesterol is part of a healthy body, but too much of it in your blood can be harmful. Eating foods that contain cholesterol (called dietary cholesterol) raises the blood cholesterol. Saturated fats and trans fats have a greater impact than dietary cholesterol in raising blood cholesterol levels. This is especially true for LDL (bad) cholesterol.

Most of the elevated cholesterol in our blood comes from eating highly refined carbohydrates and saturated fats and much less from the dietary intake cholesterol.

The cholesterol in the blood circulates in many forms. They serve different purposes. It also circulates in blood along with proteins such as low density lipoprotein (LDL cholesterol) or as high density lipoprotein (HDL cholesterol). Cholesterol and triglycerides are together called lipids. Here is a table describing the different types of cholesterol and triglycerides found in the blood.

Table of Lipid Classification

Item	Normal mg%	Borderline mg%	High mg%	Very High mg%
Total cholesterol	<200	200-239	>240	>270%
LDL cholesterol	<125	130-159	160-189	>190
HDL cholesterol	>40			
Triglycerides	<150	151-199	200-499	>500

Table of Ideal Lipid Levels in mg%

Item	Abbrev.	Action	Ideal Level	High Risk Patients
Total cholesterol	TC		<200	<160
LDL cholesterol	LDL	Bad	<100	<80
HDL cholesterol	HDL	Good	>40	>40
Triglycerides	TG		<150	<150

High risk: Patients with history of heart disease, diabetes, and vascular problems.

Total cholesterol: It represents the total cholesterol in the blood. It includes the LDL cholesterol, the HDL cholesterol, and the cholesterol bound to the triglycerides in the form of a lipoprotein complex. Note that 20% of the cholesterol traveling in the blood may be bound to the triglycerides. The total cholesterol is a reflection of the overall cholesterol in the body. If the total cholesterol in the range of 160 mg%, which some of my patients can achieve with diet and exercise, the other components will definitely be lower. The key is to work on each component of cholesterol as the approach is different for each one of them.

LDL cholesterol: LDL is the bad cholesterol made by the liver. Excess carbohydrates and fats can lead to increased levels of LDL cholesterol. The LDL cholesterol circulating freely in the body can get trapped inside the lining of the arteries, which can lead to atherosclerosis and eventually arterial blockage that can cause a heart attack and weakening of the heart muscle. According to the latest research, the desired levels of LDL (the bad cholesterol) are in the range of 60 to 80 mg%. High triglycerides tend to lead to higher LDL cholesterol levels.

Every five years the LDL cholesterol tends to go up by 5 points, unlike HDL cholesterol, which pretty much remains the same. The higher the LDL level, the greater the risk of developing heart disease. The best way to reduce the LDL cholesterol is to reduce the dietary fat intake.

HLD cholesterol: The HDL cholesterol is the good cholesterol that removes the LDL from the arterial plaques and returns it to the circulation. A small amount of the HDL comes from the diet, while the majority of the HDL cholesterol is made in the liver. The HDL cholesterol pretty much remains the same through most of your adult life. Regular exercise can raise your HDL level by a maximum of 10%. The newer cholesterol lowering pills such as statins increase HDL levels. Alcohol is known to raise HDL levels. However, there are three or four different forms of HDL in the body. It is not clear whether the rise in HDL level by alcohol really helps the heart or not. Since the benefits of alcohol are very limited compared to the enormous negative effects, I would not try excess alcohol as a means to raise your HDL level. Smoking lowers the HDL level, while weight reduction increases the HDL level.

There is no such thing as a diet rich in HDL cholesterol or a pill that can dramatically increase the HDL cholesterol. People with high blood triglycerides usually have lower HDL cholesterol levels. Female sex hormones such as estrogens raise HDL cholesterol levels. Progesterone, anabolic steroids and male sex hormones (like testosterone) also lower HDL cholesterol levels.

Cholesterol ratios: There are various ratios that measure the relationships between the HDL and total cholesterol or HDL and LDL cholesterol, among others. However, the ratios may not be a true reflection of the state when there is high triglycerides, as the total cholesterol would go up with elevated triglyceride levels. It is important to aim for the individual target levels based on the risk factors.

Triglycerides: They are a storage form of fat in the body. Triglycerides have been found to be an independent risk factor for heart disease, especially among females. High levels of triglycerides (>500 mg%) are associated with pancreatitis, which can be a serious condition at times. Many people with high triglycerides have underlying diseases or genetic disorders. Carbs raise triglyceride levels.

Dietary sources of cholesterol: Dietary cholesterol comes from meat, fish, seafood, egg yolks, butter, cheese and other dairy products made from whole milk. Foods from plants (fruits, vegetables, grains, nuts and seeds) don't contain cholesterol.

Dietary source of saturated fats: They are also an important component of the lipids, as they raise the blood cholesterol levels. Saturated fats are found in foods such as meat, lard, poultry fat, butter, cheeses and other whole-milk dairy products. Foods from some tropical plants also contain saturated fats, mainly coconut oil, palm oil, and palm kernel oil.

Trans fats are used for cooking in restaurants and most fast-food chains. Trans fats are also found in commercially baked goods and stick margarines made with partially hydrogenated vegetable oils. They're also found in some animal products such as meat and milk. Look for the words "hydrogenated fat" or "hydrogenated vegetable oil" in the ingredient list. Recently, most products sold in supermarkets may have less than 0.5 mg of trans fats. However, when you eat in restaurants, the same oil is used for several days for frying foods, and that can cause conversion of the cis fatty acids to trans fatty acids.

Dietary Treatment of Cholesterol

This will be the first approach in the treatment to lower your cholesterol. An overall reduction in calorie intake will reduce triglycerides. You also need to avoid foods such as organ meat that are rich in cholesterol. Saturated fats in the form of butter, animal fat, or cream get readily converted in the body to cholesterol. Even with the best diet control, you may only be able to drop your total cholesterol level by 25 mg%.

Also, note that you may not significantly increase the HDL or the good cholesterol by diet alone. Exercise is the only natural process by which you can increase the HDL level.

Diet can reduce triglyceride levels substantially. However, if your triglyceride levels are above 500 to 1000 mg%, you will definitely need drugs such as gemfibrozil or fenofibrate. Luckily, these drugs can reduce the triglyceride level by as much as 50 to 60%.

New cholesterol lowering spreads contain unique plant chemicals called stanols and sterol esters. They are similar in structure to cholesterol. They bind to the sites that absorb the dietary cholesterol, and thus reduce the absorption of the natural cholesterol. An average American diet contains 250 mg of plant sterols and stanols.

Spreads made with these plant stanols and sterol esters can lower LDL cholesterol by as much as 14%. They don't alter the HDL cholesterol levels. The degree of cholesterol lowering is more in people with elevated levels of cholesterol. The National Cholesterol Education Program of the U.S. National Institutes of Health recommends adding 2 grams per day of plant stanols and sterols as a general dietary plan.

Presently, two types of these products are available on the market. Take Control contains plant sterol esters. Benecol contains a plant sterol. Benecol can be used as a spread or in cooking and baking without altering the food flavor or color. It can be used in place of your regular margarine or spreads without having to worry about trans fatty acids. Take Control can be used as a spread. However, presently it is not suitable for baking or cooking. Look for Benecol or Take Control in the butter and margarine section; if your supermarket does not carry it, ask the manager to order it for you. Start enjoying your dietary fat while lowering your cholesterol levels at the same. Patients with very high levels of cholesterol may have to reduce their fat intake to less than 15% of total calories.

Each egg has 274 mg of cholesterol. Therefore, restrict whole eggs to no more than 2 per week. Instead, you could use an egg white or Egg Beaters (egg products without cholesterol). A drastic reduction in carbs, fats, and total calories will help to reduce high triglyceride levels.

I have also listed a number of supplements and natural remedies that can lower cholesterol levels by varying degrees.

Cholesterol Lowering Drugs

The HMG-CoA reductase inhibitors, commonly referred to as "statins," are considered a first-line drug therapy for the treatment of high cholesterol. HMG-CoA reductase is an enzyme made in our bodies that helps the liver produce cholesterol. Statins get in the way of that process, thus reducing the amount of cholesterol being pro-duced.

Please refer to the table below for the comparative effectiveness of commonly used statin drugs.

While each drug in this class can lower cholesterol levels, their efficacy varies from drug to drug. All of the statins lower cholesterol (and raise HDL) in a dose-dependent manner (meaning, the higher the statin dose, the greater the cholesterol reduction). However, most patients do not need the maximum dose to achieve the desired target levels.

The most common side effect seen with most of the statins is muscle aches and cramps. These drugs may cause muscle inflamma-tion and damage. However, certain studies have recommended using coenzyme Q10 (available in 100 to 200 mg doses in drug stores), which are presumed to reduce muscle-related symptoms. The second most common side effect is related to the elevation of liver enzymes. Therefore, people on statins should get their liver enzymes checked once every 3 to 6 months to ensure that the enzymes are not elevated.

If the liver enzymes are elevated, reducing the dosage might help. If that fails, switching over to a new class of drugs or a lower dose of the same drug might help.

Table of Cholesterol Lowering Drugs

Drug	Dose	TC-Dec	LDL-Dec	HDL-Inc	TG-Dec
Altocor	10-60 mg	18-29%	24-41%	9-13%	10-25%
Crestor	5-40 mg	33-46%	45-63%	8-14%	10-35%
Lescol	20-80 mg	17-27%	22-36%	3-09%	12-23%
Lescol XL	80 mg	25%	33-35%	7-11%	19-25%
Lipitor	10-80 mg	25-45%	35-60%	5-09%	19-37%
Mevacor	10-80 mg	16-34%	21-42%	2-09%	06-27%
Pravachol	10-80 mg	16-27%	22-37%	2-12%	11-24%
Zocor	5-80 mg	19-36%	26-47%	8-16%	12-33%

XL= Extended release, TC = Total cholesterol, TG =Triglycerides

Inc = Increase, Dec = Decrease

Some of the statins such as Mevacor and Zocor are available in generic forms, which can reduce your drug cost. All statins are dosed once daily, and taken at bedtime. A very important drug interaction to keep in mind is combining a statin with gemfibrozil or fenofibrate can increase the chances of muscle weakness, and rarely can cause muscle necrosis, which can be very serious.

Misconceptions About Cholesterol

Margarine instead of butter will help lower my cholesterol: Both margarine and butter are high in fat, so use both in moderation. Instead of margarines, use Benecol or Take Control, which lower cholesterol levels.

Thin people don't have to worry about high cholesterol: I have seen people who weigh more than 300 pounds who have normal cholesterol levels and lean people (under 130 lbs) who had bypass surgery for coronary artery disease. If your cholesterol level is high, it needs treatment, along with your weight, if you are overweight.

My doctor was not concerned about my cholesterol levels: Ask your doctor why he is not concerned about your cholesterol. If you can't find a satisfactory answer, seek a second opinion. The cholesterol tables mentioned above should help you to assess your risk. It pays to be an educated consumer.

If a food label says no cholesterol, does it mean it is healthy? You need to read beyond the cholesterol levels. If it has saturated fats, trans fats, and high total fat, it can be equally harmful.

Since I am on pills and my cholesterol is normal, do I still need to watch my diet? As you get less discreet with your diet, the cholesterol level will go up. I have seen patients on pills who come back with much higher cholesterol levels than what they had before taking them. On closer questioning, the patient admits eating outside the guidelines. The key is to stick to your diet.

Is cholesterol mainly a man's problem? Heart disease is the number one killer among women after the age of 50. Premenopausal women have a lesser incidence. However, it is important to pay attention to cholesterol levels, especially if you have high blood pressure and diabetes.

When is the right time to check cholesterol? The right time is if you are over the age of 40, or earlier if you have a family history of heart disease.

Lower Cholesterol Naturally

Here I have listed 22 ways to lower your cholesterol naturally.

Calorie cutback: Calorie reduction must be the initial step in your overall cholesterol reduction plan. This leads to a decline in the total and LDL cholesterol levels. Any excess calories coming from carbs, proteins, or fats, if not used for immediate energy, will eventually turn into fat that can raise your cholesterol levels. You can safely reduce your calorie intake to 1200 calories without compromising the nutritional value of your diet. Any excess calories you consume beyond that should be proportional to your physical activity and calories burned during those activities. Diabetics, no matter what type of lifestyle they are involved in, do well on 1800 calories or less per day. You can safely reduce your calorie requirements to what your body needs and not what your taste buds demand. Using my recommendation of fresh fruits, salads, beans, and grilled foods, you can eat normal foods and lose weight at the same time. The sugar in sweets very quickly spikes triglycerides in people. Avoid fruit juices, soda, pastries, pies, candy, cookies, starchy foods, and sweet desserts.

Dietary cholesterol: If you eat one whole egg on one day (one egg has 274 mg of cholesterol), try to avoid or limit other sources of dietary cholesterol on that day. You could eat 2 to 3 egg whites or egg substitutes per day in place of whole eggs. Drastically reduce your consumption of fried foods, saturated fats, chicken skin, meat with visible fat, and spreads that have trans fatty acids. Avoid eating baked goods (like muffins, cookies and cakes) that are rich in carbs, fats, and cholesterol. Make sure your meat choices are lean and no more than 4 to 6 ounces per meal. Select cholesterol-free vegetarian choices in place of meats for one of your daily meals.

Fiber: Since fiber can lower your LDL cholesterol level by 10 to 15%, include foods high in fiber such as green leafy vegetables, whole grains, and beans in your daily meals. Soluble fiber is also found in fiber supplements or in fruits such as apples, grapes, and citrus fruits. The fiber in these foods helps lower total cholesterol levels and often raises HDL levels. It is believed that fiber binds to cholesterol in the small intestine and prevents cholesterol absorption into the bloodstream, thus reducing cholesterol levels. You need to consume at least 30 grams of fiber per day. One example is psyllium, a fiber source that is seen primarily in Iran or India. It is primarily used in traditional herbal medicines and is a common ingredient in bulk laxative products as well. A study of psyllium showed that its consumption in the form of supplements lowered LDL cholesterol levels. The same study showed LDL level improvement in both children and adults. This benefit of psyllium is believed to come from its soluble fiber component. Another example of a rich source of fiber is oat bran, a common breakfast staple. In one study, participants eating 2 ounces of oat bran per day showed a 16% reduction in LDL levels and a 15% increase in HDL levels. Oat bran and barley have soluble fibers known as beta-glucans that lower cholesterol levels.

Body weight: Obesity is a major cause of high triglyceride levels. If you are overweight, lose weight with regular exercise and by reducing your total calorie intake.

Red wines: Red wines such as Cabernet, Sauvignon, Merlot, and Pinot Noir contain antioxidants that slow down the oxidation of LDL cholesterol, which reduces the amount of LDL deposited in arterial plaques. Limit your intake of red wine to no more than 1 to 2 glasses per day.

Orange juice: In one study conducted at the University of Western Ontario in Canada, 25 students drank orange juice every day for a 4-week period and had a 21% increase in their HDL levels. The rise in HDL was thought to be related to the flavonoid (an antioxidant) in the orange juice.

Beans: Kidney and red beans are a wonderful choice for raising HDL. The low-glycemic index carbohydrates in these foods cause less profound insulin spikes. People who consume foods rich in low-glycemic carbohydrates have higher HDL levels.

Fish: Fish rich in omega-3 fatty acids, eaten several times a week, can raise your HDL level. Sardines, salmon, sea bass, herring, mackerel and tuna fall in this category. If you do not like to eat fish, fish-oil capsules can be used as a supplement.

Olive oil: Olive oil, which is high in monounsaturated fatty acids, has been shown to lower blood cholesterol. Extra-virgin olive oil is suggested to be better than other varieties. Include 1 to 2 teaspoons of olive oil with each meal.

Cholesterol lowering spreads: Spreads made with plant stanols and sterols esters lower cholesterol to a greater extent in people with elevated cholesterol than in those with normal cholesterol levels. These sterols trick your intestine into thinking they are cholesterol. When the intestine tries to absorb them, it is not able to, therefore blocking actual cholesterol from being absorbed. The National Cholesterol Education Program of the National Institutes of Health recommends adding 2 grams per day of plant stanols and sterols into a general dietary plan. Presently, two types of these products are available on the market. Take Control contains plant sterol esters, and Benecol contains a plant sterol. Benecol can be used as a spread or in cooking and baking without altering the food flavor or color. Because it does not contain any trans fatty acids, it is a safe substitute for all other margarines and spreads. Take Control can be used as a spread. However, it is not presently suitable for baking or cooking. Switch your normal margarine or butter choices to Benecol or Take Control products that are specifically designed to help reduce cholesterol.

Onions: Some research suggests that eating one half of a raw onion per day may raise HDL levels by as much as 30%.

Soy products: Soy products have been shown to lower total cholesterol, LDL cholesterol, and triglycerides, and to raise HDL cholesterol. To achieve the desired results (15 to 25% reduction in cholesterol), you have to consume at least 25 grams of soy protein per day. Soy protein is available in numerous forms such as fresh soybeans, protein bars, shakes, milk and tofu.

Nuts: Nuts such as almonds and walnuts have high amounts of monounsaturated or polyunsaturated fatty acids that help lower cholesterol. Researchers at Loma Linda University found that a diet containing pecans not only lowered total and LDL cholesterol levels significantly, but also helped to maintain desirable HDL cholesterol levels. Another study found that the Mediterranean style diet, which includes walnuts, lowers cholesterol.

Trans fatty acids: Avoid eating foods such as French fries, cookies, cakes and many of the fried fast foods that are rich in trans fatty acids. They function as saturated fats and raise your cholesterol levels.

Minimize carbohydrates: Minimize your consumption of simple carbohydrates—sugar, flour, potatoes, white rice, etc.—because your body can turn them into fat and cholesterol. Blood sugar is spiked by eating carbohydrates, which also lower your HDL cholesterol level.

Smoking cessation: According to a study from Vanderbilt, people who quit smoking experienced a rise in their HDL levels by seven points.

Royal jelly: One way to help reduce your cholesterol levels while you quit smoking may be to have a little royal jelly. Surprisingly, this has been noticed to lower cholesterol levels by reducing some of the cholesterol-elevating effects of nicotine.

Natural supplements: Having several different avenues for lowering cholesterol is important because the causes of high cholesterol levels vary greatly from person to person. Natural remedies such as guggul, pantethine, policosanol, curcumin, and beta-sitosterol are just a few supplements that are easily available at a low cost compared to prescribed drugs.

Guggul: A gum resin from the mukul myrrh tree known as guggul has been shown to lower cholesterol levels. In one trial, the researchers who compared guggal to clofibrate, a cholesterol-lowering drug, noted that the average fall in total cholesterol was slightly greater in the guggul group. The HDL cholesterol level also rose in 60% of people in the guggul group.

Pantothine: Some people who have taken pantothine, a naturally occurring substance (one of the B vitamins), have noticed an increase in their HDL levels.

Policosanol: It is a dietary supplement, a mixture of alcohols isolated from Cuban sugarcane wax. It inhibits cholesterol formation in the liver. One study showed a reduction in total cholesterol levels by 17% and LDL cholesterol levels by 28%, and an increase in HDL cholesterol levels by 28% in those people who took policosanol compared to those who did not take it.

Curcumin: This product, commonly found in turmeric, reduces cholesterol levels by interfering with intestinal cholesterol uptake, increasing the conversion of cholesterol into bile acids, and increasing the excretion of bile acids.

Niacin: This naturally occurring substance (one of the B vitamins) lowers total cholesterol levels, raises HDL levels (as much as 15 to 30%), and reduces triglyceride levels (as much as 50%). It comes in 500 mg tablets and can be taken 2 to 3 times a day. Combining niacin with vitamin B6 can minimize facial flushing, a common side effect of niacin resulting from blood vessel dilatation. Niacin combined with inositol has been shown to cause less flushing.

Chromium: Chromium supplements have been shown to increase HDL cholesterol levels by an average of nearly 6 points (a 16% increase), leading to a 20% reduction in the heart attack risk.

Calcium citrate: Taking one gram of calcium daily (as the citrate) has been shown to lower LDL cholesterol levels by 6% and increase HDL cholesterol levels by 7%.

Vitamins B and C: B vitamins also lower LDL levels by decreasing the rate at which LDL is oxidized. Only oxidized LDL cholesterol can get into the arterial plaques. In addition, vitamin C has been noted to slightly reduce cholesterol levels.

Carnitine: This natural supplement also has been shown to increase HDL levels.

Coenzyme Q10: It has been noted to reduce total cholesterol levels. It has also improved the heart function of patients with heart failure.

Garlic: This little plant bulb that lowers blood pressure has also been widely studied for its cholesterol lowering properties.

Grapeseed extract: Another unusual cholesterol lowering supplement, this has also been noted to reduce total serum cholesterol levels.

Flaxseeds: Flaxseeds provide alpha-linolenic acid, a polyunsaturated fatty acid that has been shown to lower cholesterol, while also providing needed soluble fiber. The polyunsaturated fatty acids in flaxseed include omega-3 fatty acids that stabilize the arterial lining membranes.

Red yeast rice: This Chinese red yeast rice comes from a fermenting yeast called *Monascus purpureus* that grows on red rice. Red yeast rice has been noted to have a substance similar to the statin prescription drugs that lower cholesterol. *Monascus purpureus* also inhibits the action of HMG-CoA reductase. Presently, the U.S. Food and Drug Administration (FDA) classifies red yeast rice as a dietary supplement. Some studies of red yeast rice have shown it to reduce total cholesterol levels by 16%, LDL cholesterol by 21%, and triglycerides by 24%, while increasing HDL by 14%. It is available as 500 to 600 mg capsules that can be taken 2 to 4 times daily. However, just as with the statins, red yeast rice also has been shown to affect the liver. Hence, you need to have liver tests done if you are taking the pills for a long period.

Grapefruit juice: When grapefruit or grapefruit juice is taken with HMG-CoA reductase inhibitors (such as Lipitor, Zocor, Crestor and Pravachol), it enhances the effect of the medications. It also causes a significant increase in the blood levels of the drug, leading to a greater risk of serious side effects or liver damage. Because red yeast rice appears to act in much the same way as these cholesterol lowering drugs, it would be wise to avoid grapefruit, grapefruit juice, and other grapefruit products (such as marmalade) while taking red yeast rice.

Chapter 15

Smoking
If you've had it, just say no!

Hazards of Smoking

If you smoke one pack of cigarettes a day, you are investing roughly $3285 (365 x $9.00) per year in the tobacco industry. This $3285 yearly investment, with compound interest, could spiral to over $200,000 during the next 30 years. That does not include the extra $50,000 to $100,000 you may have to pay in medical costs directly related to your smoking habit. The tobacco industry spends $5000 of your money every minute promoting and advertising its products. Well, I am merely trying to inform you of your huge investment in this multibillion-dollar industry. You are a major shareholder in this deadly enterprise if you persist in smoking. Let us look at a list of some of the returns on your investment in the tobacco industry.

The dangerous and unwanted effects of smoking: The American Lung Association reports that 430,000 deaths each year are directly related to smoking, with heart attacks accounting for the largest percent. In fact, cigarette smoking accounts for more deaths yearly than those from AIDS, drug abuse, car accidents, and homicides combined! Smoking not only *increases* your risk of painful death, but it also *decreases* your lifespan. Each time you light a cigarette, you have chosen to die 13 minutes earlier. Cigarette smoking, considered a form of drug dependency, damages your heart, lungs, and blood vessels.

Nicotine addiction: Cigarette smoke contains around 4300 chemicals, the most dangerous of which is nicotine, a very addictive substance. Nicotine acutely increases your heart rate, breathing rate, blood pressure, and the volume of blood pumped by your heart. It also increases the blood clotting tendency and the heart muscle's oxygen requirement. In addition, it adversely affects the brain and nervous system and directly influences certain brain cell receptors that regulate one's mood, alertness, concentration, and refluxes. Nicotine increases the brain's alpha activity, leading to a sense of relaxation or even alertness. It can reach your brain within seven seconds after inhalation of cigarette smoke. Therefore, nicotine may act as both a stimulant or a sedative. Since the endorphins released by nicotine provide a feeling of tranquility, many people smoke to relieve their stress, anxiety, or loneliness.

However, nicotine is an addictive chemical. Soon, larger and larger doses of nicotine are needed to satisfy the craving. Tolerance to this chemical develops very rapidly. When you smoke a cigarette, the nicotine level gradually goes up in your blood. About 30 minutes after finishing a cigarette, the nicotine level comes down, inducing a craving for more nicotine. As your tolerance to nicotine builds up, you will seek larger doses to satisfy your desire.

When you decide to quit smoking, be aware of various nicotine withdrawal symptoms. Anxiety, headaches, mood changes, upset stomach, sleep deprivation, dizziness, tremors, and appetite fluctuations are common manifestations of nicotine withdrawal. Although these withdrawal symptoms may last for days, weeks, or even months, the benefits of nicotine withdrawal and quitting smoking far outweigh these minor but annoying symptoms.

Heart problems: Smoking is the number two risk factor for heart disease, after cholesterol. Smokers have twice the heart disease risk of nonsmokers and have fewer chances of surviving a heart attack than nonsmokers. Chronic smokers have lower levels of HDL cholesterol (the good cholesterol). Smoking also causes major vascular problems. Carbon monoxide, a major byproduct of smoking, reduces the amount of oxygen available for your heart and other organs. Smoking also promotes disproportionate fat distribution around the waist (a greater waist-to-hip ratio) that increases your heart disease risk.

Lung diseases: Smoking is the principal cause of chronic lung disease. Smokers have a 10-fold increased risk of lung cancer and a 20-fold increase in emphysema compared with non-smokers. Unfortunately, any lung damage caused by smoking is permanent. Parents must avoid smoking around their young children since the children are more susceptible to lung diseases resulting from cigarette smoke. Infants up to 2 years old who are exposed to parental smoke have a much greater risk of developing bronchitis and pneumonia.

Blood clotting and arterial problems: Smoking adversely alters the platelet function in the blood, leading to increased blood clotting. Generally, during the final stages of a heart attack, a blood clot forms at the site of a critically narrowed artery, causing a complete occlusion, or blockage, of an artery. It also increases the hardening process in the lining of blood vessels supplying the brain and the legs. This process, known as atherosclerosis, consists of a thickening of the arterial inner lining, fat and cholesterol deposition beneath the arterial inner lining, and smooth muscle cell growth. Over time, arteries damaged by atherosclerosis lose their elasticity and become increasingly stiff and narrow. Smoking can also lead to arterial blockages in the legs, resulting in peripheral arterial disease. This condition causes intermittent pain while walking, a condition known as claudication. It also leads to poor circulation, and, in a worst case scenario, could lead to eventual loss of a limb. Diabetes compounds the smoking-related vascular problems.

Women and children: Although the smoking incidence has been steadily declining over the past few years among men, it has been rapidly rising among women and teenagers. Death rates among women from smoking-related lung disease are reaching those of men. This smoking trend among women is strange since women smokers have two-and-a-half times the risk of stroke than non-smokers. Female smokers also have lower levels of estrogen and have a greater risk of osteoporosis. In addition, they are more likely to experience an earlier menopause. Lady smokers on birth control pills increase their heart disease risk several-fold. Pregnant women smokers have higher rates of miscarriage and of stillborn and premature babies. They are also likely to face more pregnancy-related complications. Their children also face many dangers from their mothers' smoking habit. Infants born to smokers are more likely to die of crib death than the babies of non-smokers. In addition, second-hand smoke is very harmful to children. From 150,000 to 300,000 children suffer each year from bronchitis and other respiratory diseases because of second-hand smoke.

Oral cancer: The use of smokeless tobacco is rapidly rising, especially among school-age males. Chewing tobacco or using moist snuff increases your chances of getting oral cancer. These products contain cancer-causing nitrosamines at levels hundreds of times greater than those legally allowed for certain foods.

Arthritis: Arthritis is another painful problem often suffered by smokers. In fact, male smokers are almost 8 times more likely to develop rheumatoid arthritis than non-smokers, and ex-smokers have 4 times the risk of developing this crippling disease. Exposure to tobacco smoke triggers rheumatoid factor production, which in combination with male hormones, contributes to the exacerbation of arthritis and its symptoms.

According to the American Lung Association, the side-stream smoke coming from the tips of burning cigarettes completely escapes the cigarette filters and directly enters the air. This type of smoke contains more harmful compounds—tar, nicotine, carbon monoxide, etc.—than the mainstream smoke exhaled by smokers. Most of the smoke filling restaurants and nightclubs is comprised of this harmful second-hand smoke.

Low-tar cigarettes: There is evidence that low-tar and low-nic-otine cigarettes aren't any better than regular cigarettes in reducing heart disease risk. Because of the addictive nature of nicotine, try-ing to switch to a low-nicotine cigarette generally results in a more frequent consumption of these low-nicotine cigarettes to make up for the decreased nicotine supply. People who smoke low-nicotine cigarettes are more likely to inhale more deeply when they smoke.

Stinking odor: A preacher once told a friend of mine, "Jeffery, smoking may not send you to hell, but the cigarette smell sure makes you feel like you have returned from one."

Smoking leaves an unpleasant smell on your skin, clothes, and breath that remains on you long after you have smoked the cigarette or left the smoke-filled restaurant. However, as a smoker, you may be unable to recognize the odor because of the destruction of the smell receptors in the inner lining of your nose as a result of long-term smoking.

Benefits of Smoking Cessation

Following the 1986 Surgeon General's report on the deadly effects of smoking, more and more states and local laws have restricted or eliminated smoking practices in public places. Almost all hospitals have now adopted a no-smoking policy. All domestic airlines throughout the country have banned smoking on their flights. Some states have even banned smoking in bars and nightclubs! An increasing number of private companies are rewarding their employees for adapting a smoke-free policy for their workplace.

Weight gain following smoking cessation is a recognized phenomenon. Sometimes, it is used as an excuse for replacing a smoking habit with an equally bad eating habit. A modest 5 to 10 pound weight gain is noted in 65% of people who quit smoking. On the other hand, if you gain 50 to 75 pounds after smoking cessation, you'd better seek some other explanation for that weight gain. Immediately following smoking cessation, avoid overindulgence in calories, inactivity, and preoccupying your mind with the loss of your beloved friend, the cigarette. Women or formerly heavy smokers tend to gain slightly more weight; but with proper guidance and support, even these high-risk smokers can limit their weight gain to fewer than 2 pounds.

One year after you quit smoking, your cardiac-related health risks reduce to the level seen among non-smokers. After 2 years, your stroke risk returns to the normal level. Women who stop smoking notice an increase in their HDL cholesterol (good cholesterol) by

7 mg% within a couple of months. That is not a bad deal, especially if you have been smoking for the past 10 or 20 years.

Other benefits include the return of your senses of smell and taste, easier breathing, and normal digestion of foods. That nagging smoker's cough also disappears. It becomes easier for you to control your bronchitis or emphysema symptoms. Overall, you will enjoy better health, feel more energetic, and live longer. Consider also all the money you will save from reduced trips to the hospital because of smoking-related health problems. How about the co-payment cost savings? Now, that is a definite reason to quit smoking!

One final thought: You could use the money you saved from smoking cessation to put one of your family members or even yourself through medical school to become a doctor. If you do not intend to become a doctor, just donate that savings to the American Heart Association, the American Lung Association, or the American Cancer society. You may say, "I don't want to be a doctor, so why should I give my money to others?" My only reply would be "Well, it is better than using it to fill the tobacco industry's coffins!"

Smoking Cessation Resources

In the United States, 1.5 million people quit smoking each year. Although this number might sound huge, in reality, an additional 50 million adults could benefit from smoking cessation. Smoking cessation is not an easy step to take, especially if you have been smoking for many years. It will take a lot of earnest work and determination to kick a habit that has seized most of your life.

Do not try to quit smoking merely to impress your doctor or your spouse. That effort will be short-lived. The decision to quit smoking has to be an unconditional resolve stemming from your heart and soul. Making that decision will be one of the most important steps in your life. Therefore, be sure to highlight and etch in your mind the benefits you will enjoy by kicking the habit, which will give you the enthusiasm and the incentive to keep up with your long-term goal.

Smoking cessation strengthens your confidence in yourself and paves your path toward joyful, heart healthy living. When you quit smoking, you are saying good-bye to your destructive smoking habit, nicotine addiction, and repulsive smoke smell.

At this time, it is essential that you develop new habits and activities to replace your old smoking habit. These changes demand time, patience, commitment, and adaptation. It is not as simple as merely listening to a motivational or hypnosis audiotape on smoking termination to reprogram your life. Although only hearing a lecture may work in some exceptional cases, you will have to mobilize substantial effort to permanently conquer this deadly habit.

Preparation: Once you have decided to quit smoking for good, set a date for totally dropping the habit. Eliminate from your home everything related to your smoking habit: ashtray, lighter, matches, and, of course, your cigarettes. Tell all your friends that you are going to quit. Once you make your decision public, you cannot go back on your promise. This allows for accountability with those who care about you. When a cigarette craving suddenly attacks you during the day, rely on small amounts of low-calorie snacks, walking, or a hot shower to overcome the urge. Never allow overindulgence in food to trade places with your smoking habit. Post a big sign over your refrigerator reminding you not to touch that ice cream or cheesecake, especially during periods of nicotine withdrawal pains. Better yet, get rid of any high-caloric temptations from your house. Put the "Out of Sight, Out of Mind" psychology to work in your favor.

Support: Encourage your family and friends to help you quit smoking. That means they also have to kick the smoking habit if they want to support you. When you are trying to quit, you will not make any progress if your spouse fills up your living room, bedroom, and lungs with your favorite cigarette smoke. If your smoking friends do not want to cooperate, then it is time to make some new friends. (Avoid those who want to replace your smoking habit with alcohol.) Establish a friendship with people who also are trying to quit the smoking habit so you can exchange ideas, thoughts, and feelings.

Behavior modification: Cultivate a habit of doing something enjoyable every day to counteract the cigarette urge. Drink a lot of water and other fluids. Use medications or nicotine supplements under the supervision of a qualified physician. Take long walks or bicycle rides and carry sugarless gum with you or munch on celery sticks. If you get the urge to smoke, resist it — especially during the first 5 minutes. The first 2 to 5 minutes will always be the toughest. Remind yourself that you have made a promise to yourself, your family, and friends that you *will* quit the smoking habit.

Approaches: There are several approaches to smoking cessation, and different techniques highlight different aspects. Some programs cost a substantial sum of money. Whatever program you choose, make sure that it has worked effectively for many others in the past. Do not hesitate to ask program representatives for statistics and references. You do not want to become a bitter statistic in their program. If you are not satisfied with the program for any reason, contact the local branch of the American Lung Association for the programs they support. They have several well-tested programs for those who want to quit smoking.

I have listed below some common smoking cessation programs, discussing their success rates, benefits, and drawbacks. I hope this list will provide you with useful information in deciding which program might be best suitable for you.

Group sessions: The American Lung Association has many comprehensive educational and smoking cessation programs for individuals, workplaces, pregnant mothers, schools, teens, and children exposed to second-hand smoke. Please visit *www.lungusa.org* for information and instructions on ordering these invaluable tools to help you cultivate a tobacco-free life. The most popular smoking cessation program, *Freedom From Smoking*, is available for individuals, schools, workplaces, and instructors.

Nicotine patches: Nicotine patches by themselves are not a cure for your smoking habit. They simply provide the nicotine you are craving in a patch form while you are enrolled in a smoking cessation program. Unlike the nicotine from smoking that passes almost immediately into your bloodstream, the nicotine in the patch may take up to 3 hours to reach your bloodstream. These patches resemble large bandages that you wear on a daily basis. Nicotine patches differ in their nicotine contents, and the manner in which they release the drug.

However, the patch approach does have its downfalls. Most smokers give up patches because of the slow nicotine delivery by the patches, which does not help to curb their nicotine urge. They also do not develop patch dependency for the same reason. Each patch may cost as much as a whole pack of cigarettes. In addition, I have seen people smoking while they are on the patch at the same time. Now, guess what happens when you do that? You are getting double the nicotine dose. No wonder you feel better on a combination of a patch and cigarettes. It may convince your spouse at first that you are trying, but, in reality, you will never be able to kick your smoking habit this way. If you cannot stop smoking, you are advised by pharmaceutical companies not to use the nicotine patches. Some people cannot wear the patches because of skin irritation or profuse sweating problems. Headaches, dizziness, vivid dreams, weakness, and upset stomach are other common side effects.

Nicotine gum: When you chew this gum, set amounts of nicotine are released, which reduces your urge to smoke. Nicotine from the gum takes several minutes to reach the brain. Nicotine makes it way into your blood through the cheek lining, as you chew the gum a few times to break it into small bits and park the broken bits between your gum and cheek. This gum is available in 2 mg doses (for those who smoke less than 24 cigarettes per day) and 4 mg doses (for those who smoke more than 24 cigarettes per day). You must stop smoking when you are using nicotine gum. Do not eat or drink for 15 minutes while using the gum, and do not mix it with saliva and swallow it, as it may upset your stomach. Some smokers may have to chew 10 to 15 sticks of gum per day (maximum 30 per day). If you do not have good results after 30 days of use, consult with your physician. This gum is available only by prescription and is intended as only a temporary aid for smokers trying to quit. It can be used in conjunction with other programs to reduce your nicotine withdrawal symptoms.

Nicotine lozenge: This new product, available as a hard candy, releases nicotine slowly while it dissolves in your mouth. However, biting or chewing it releases more nicotine, resulting in indigestion and/or heartburn. Therefore, avoid eating or drinking during this period. It is available in 2 mg or 4 mg doses. Do not use more than 20 lozenges (doses) per day. The lozenge may stay in your mouth for 30 minutes. The common side effects are teeth and gum soreness, indigestion, and throat irritation.

Nicotine nasal spray: Resembling an ordinary nasal spray, the nicotine spray delivers nicotine more rapidly than most other nicotine products, which is an attractive feature to many smokers. You deliver two sprays to each nostril. A maximum of 5 doses per hour or 40 doses total per day is recommended. The most common side effects are nose and throat irritation.

Nicotine inhaler: Resembling a cigarette, this plastic cylinder with a cartridge delivers nicotine when you puff on it. However, the nicotine is delivered into your mouth and not into your lungs. Available only by prescription, each cartridge delivers up to 400 puffs of nicotine vapor. You have to take at least 80 puffs to get the nicotine effect of one cigarette. You achieve the best results by frequent and continuous puffing for 20 minutes. One cartridge lasts for 20 minutes and delivers 4 mg of nicotine (equal to 2 cigarettes). The maximum suggested dose is 16 cartridges per day. Side effects include mouth irritation.

The cold turkey approach: Most of the people who I treat for heart attacks immediately quit smoking during their hospital stays in the intensive care unit. Personally, I think it is great that they quit smoking after having a heart attack and stay smoke-free for the rest of their lives, and I wish others could do the same. However, I do not want you to wait until you get a heart attack before you beef up your willpower to quit smoking. If you have the willpower to quit after a heart attack, then you must have had that willpower all along. You just did not feel it was necessary to exercise that power. It is the fear of a second heart attack that shifts your thinking into a higher state.

Self-help methods: Many books, audiotapes, videotapes, and DVDs are available to help you quit smoking. The American Lung Association also can provide you with a list of materials that covers everything from understanding your habits to changing your lifestyle. Self-help approaches may not be as effective as the planned programs, where you get the motivation and support group. However, they do provide you with valuable knowledge and information that will benefit you whether you try to quit on your own or with a group program.

The American Cancer Society has programs for individuals, workplaces, and the community. The American Heart Association supplies brochures and videotapes. The American Lung Association offers programs such as:

- Freedom from Smoking
- Not-on-Tobacco
- Tips for Parents
- Quitter in You

In one study, researchers found that people who followed a structured smoking cessation group program had a much higher success rate compared to those who did not. They also noted a 50% overall reduction in death rates over a period of 14.5 years among those who were enrolled in the smoking cessation group program. The authors concluded the ongoing group support and behavior modifications played an important role in sustaining smoking cessation, which may be difficult to achieve on one's own.

Hypnosis: Hypnosis has been found useful for certain smokers when administered by a qualified and trained hypnotherapist. It is even more effective when the training is spread over several weeks. However, consider the cost of such programs. If you are not easily hypnotized, this may get very expensive, and you may not get the best benefit from this approach. If you do want to follow this approach, make sure the therapy is provided by a psychiatrist, psychologist, or social worker with experience and a good track record.

Acupuncture: Acupuncture is based on an ancient Chinese practice. Fine needles are inserted into specific places on your body where nerve connections are present to achieve certain responses by your body. Yet, there is no sound evidence that this technique helps people quit smoking. It may only serve as a "placebo effect" for the smoker who is trying to overcome the smoking habit and nicotine addiction. This method is often not sufficient by itself and requires other smoking cessation programs to be practiced at the same time. In addition to acupuncture, you likely need motivation, education, group support, and counseling.

The electric shock and rapid smoking methods: The rapid smoking method is where you inhale smoke every 6 seconds until you cannot tolerate smoke anymore. This effect may take up to 4 to 6 minutes to occur on your first try. Try this once or twice during a session. You may have to repeat this process up to 10 times before you begin to feel nauseated whenever you think of lighting another cigarette. If you have significant heart or lung problems, this smoking cessation approach may prove very dangerous. As always, consult with your physician before you try this method.

The electric shock method delivers small electrical shocks to people each time they light a cigarette. This is used to remind the smoker that he should avoid lighting that cigarette. However, most people tend to remove the batteries from the devices to avoid the shock. Neither of these two methods is popular today.

Over-the-counter products: Among all the products available, Nicocure, Nicozan, and NutraQuit are most popular. Their popularity is based on high overall effectiveness, low side effects, guarantee, and a high success rate.

Non-nicotine pill: Bupropion hydrochloride (Zyban), a prescription medicine originally approved for depression, has been found useful for smoking cessation (150 to 300 mg/day). It is started one week before you quit and then continued for 7 weeks while you engage in a smoking cessation group program. The usefulness of this drug beyond 7 to 8 weeks is unknown. If you are not successful by that time, then you are advised to discontinue the drug.

Smoking cessation success rates: As a final note, I do want to mention that even with the best program, the one-year quit rate is around 25% to 40%. That means that more than half of the people who try to quit go right back to smoking. If you want to quit smoking, you need a program that not only helps you to quit the smoking habit, but also to stay smoke-free. You need a program that provides you with appropriate guidelines that will last for years, supplying you with energy and vigor until you have eliminated your cigarette need. The determination has to come from within you.

Do not be discouraged if you are not successful on your first try. Refuse to give up. The only thing you should give up is your smoking habit. Do not quit until the smoking habit quits you. The single most important factor in the smoking cessation path will be your determination. The rest will follow.

When you enroll in a program, consider the following points:

- Is it the right plan for you?
- Is the location convenient for you?
- Are the staff well trained and encouraging?
- Do they provide follow-up support?
- Do they stand by their program?
- What is their success rate?
- What does their program cost?
- Who supports their program?
- What are the likely chances of your sticking with the program?

Internet Resources:

American Heart Association www.americanheart.org

American lung association www.lungusa.org/

Surgeon General www.surgeongeneral.gov/tobacco

Quit smoking www.quitnet.com/

CDC www.cdc.gov/tobacco/

Stop smoking center www.stopsmokingcenter.net/

In the Internet era, be aware of people disguised as experts trying to push their products. Instead, review information from the reputable sources such as the American Lung Association or the American Heart Association. As always, consult with your physician before carrying out any plan, since your physician is most familiar with your complete medical history.

Notes:

Chapter 16

Exercise Part-1

Exercise is the key to your Wellness

Before you read this, I expect you may be wondering, "What's in it for me?" So without wasting one more precious moment of your non-refundable time, let me tell you about the grand benefits of enrolling yourself in a regular exercise program.

Benefits of Exercise

Zig Ziglar, one of the nation's foremost motivational speakers, once said, "If you don't like the way you look, you are not stuck with you. You can change the way you look by changing what goes into your mind." I would like to expand on that theme and say, "If you don't like the way you look, feel, or act, don't worry about it." You can change the way you look, feel, or act by enrolling yourself in a regular exercise program.

Looks: There are two kinds of looks. Someone may walk up to you and say, "You look marvelously great," and really mean it. On the other hand, he may say, "That dress looks gorgeous on you." You have no idea what he means by that. Well, you don't have to listen to those comments if you enroll in a regular exercise program.

When you exercise regularly, you can trim off years of over-hanging front and side effects that have been robbing your mind and self-esteem. In addition, regular exercise can tone your muscles and enhance your gracious silhouette. For example, if you start walking for 30 minutes a day, without changing anything else, at the end of one year you will have lost 14 pounds. Later, I will show you how you can easily lose one pound per week with regular exercise, with very little modification to your regular eating habits.

Feelings: If you don't have a million dollars, you can't feel like someone who has a million dollars. If you have a million dollars, you may be too busy working on your second million dollars. Right after you finish a 30-minute exercise, you may feel like someone who has a million dollars. That sensation of euphoria, resulting from the release of endorphins, lasts for several hours after the exercise is over. Exercise also reduces your anxiety, tension, and stress. When you are jogging at a speed of four to five miles per hour, you have no time to blame others or pick a fight with someone else.

Acting: It is for those who can't exercise. Regular exercise improves your muscle strength, increases your stamina, decreases your fatigue, and improves your body weight. As a result, you can quit pretending and start performing better.

Cardiovascular benefits: Regular exercise improves your heart function. Trained athletes have a lower heart rate response to the same level of exercise than untrained athletes. Exercise is the only natural way to increase your HDL cholesterol (the good part of the cholesterol that removes the cholesterol deposits from blocked arteries). It also improves the collateral circulation (small new channels that carry extra blood to the heart muscle) to your heart. This improves your chances of surviving a second heart attack. It improves the oxygen used by the skeletal muscles, and as a result, the heart has to work less for a given workload.

Other benefits: Exercise helps to lower your blood pressure. Frequently, regular exercise and weight control can reduce your need for the medicines used to control your blood pressure or occasionally, eliminate the need for medicines. Exercise also reduces the insulin requirement in diabetics.

Risks of Exercise

Muscles and joints: Erma Bombeck said that she hates to get involved in an activity where there is an ambulance waiting at the finish line. You don't have to visit the ski slopes to sustain a torn ligament or a sprained ankle. Try running a 100 meter dash in hot, humid, die-hard weather, especially if you have never exercised before. You can develop severe muscle cramps that can result in lingering pain through long summer days. This will convince you that exercise is hazardous to your delicate lifestyle and health. Of course, when you want to learn and experience everything about exercise in one weekend, I sympathize with your muscles and joints. On the other hand, if you start your exercise program with a step-by-step approach as described later in this chapter, you don't have to worry about painful cramps or busted joints.

Heat exhaustion: The symptoms of heat exhaustion include low temperature, dizziness, headache, confusion, and nausea. Heat stroke is a more serious condition that is associated with dizziness, thirst, nausea, headache, and muscle cramps. The drenching sweating stops and the body temperature rises quickly. You can avoid both of these problems by drinking plenty of fluids and wearing cool and light clothes.

Heart attack: Some people are afraid that they might have a heart attack during exercise. The interesting point is that people have had heart attacks during sleep, during the early hours of the morning, in the evenings, and at rest. Some people have had heart attacks while watching TV. It's not clear that exercise can precipitate a heart attack. On the contrary, regular exercise should lower the risk of having a heart attack. However, if you have severe unsuspected heart disease, and you relentlessly push yourself beyond your limit, then you may be asking for trouble.

If you have congenital heart disease (birth defects such as aortic valve narrowing) or irregular heart rhythms, you may be at an increased risk of serious problems resulting from sustained and vigorous exercise. Therefore, you should consult your physician before you enroll yourself in a regular exercise program.

Money: If you get too carried away by the passions of exercise, you may end spending a fortune on exercise gear and club memberships. However, when your early enthusiasm wears off and your mind wanders into the wilderness again, your expensive exercise gear may die a slow death while collecting dust and mold in your garage. It may even become a constant source of irritation among family members. Consider this before you sweat a great deal of fortune.

Exercise Myths

It's too tiring: A lady once said, "Doc, I ache all over." Dr. Charles W. Jarvis, a humorist, said, "Ma'am, those are the muscles you have never used." If you realize it takes 72 muscles perfectly coordinated to utter a single word, you can imagine how many muscles are involved in jogging or skiing.

You can expect to feel some soreness in your muscles at the beginning of your exercise program. However, if you get tired easily following a routine exercise, you need to be concerned about medical problems such as a heart condition or low blood count. In such cases, I recommend that you consult with your doctor. Regular exercise also increases your stamina and strength, which can reduce your fatigue and tiredness.

It takes too much time: People often say, "It takes too much time." I ask, "Compared to what?" Thirty minutes of exercise three times a week amounts to one and one half hours per week. There are 24 hours in a day. If you were to multiply 24 by 7, that gives you 168 hours in a week. Therefore, you don't have to belong to an accountants' club to realize the time you spend exercising is less than one percent of the time in any given week. It is not the lack of time; it is the lack of planning that robs your life and time. Therefore, if you carefully plan your exercise and include that in your daily activity schedule, it will only be a matter of days or weeks before it becomes a part of your daily life.

Don't forget that 50 percent of your working time is spent on earnings that go toward paying some kind of taxes. Now, let me ask you, "Which one do you like better? Exercising for an hour and a half per week to maintain your health and well-being, or working for half the time to pay your taxes?" I bet you're glad I asked this question.

All exercises are the same: Not all physical activities produce cardiac fitness. Sustained exercises involving large groups of muscles, such as jogging, jumping rope, running, or skiing produce the maximum cardiovascular benefits. They also help you burn many calories. Tennis, handball, and basketball also produce cardiac conditioning, but to a lesser degree. Besides, these exercises also have to be performed for a much longer duration of time. Others, such as baseball, football, or softball, do not provide any significant cardiovascular conditioning.

Older people need less exercise: As you get older, there is a tendency for you to be less active. You also lose muscle mass each year. Therefore, to maintain your muscle mass and physical fitness, you need the same amount of exercise as a younger individual. You can engage in different types of exercises depending upon your age and physical characteristics.

You have to be an athlete: You don't have to be an athlete to engage in a regular exercise program. In fact, many people who were discouraged during their school years because they were not able to compete with their peers in sports have discovered that regular exercise is something they not only can perform very easily, but also can enjoy.

Consult your physician before you enroll yourself in a regular exercise program. Your physician can do a complete examination and make sure you do not have serious medical problems that might interfere with your exercise. Your physician can also prescribe the right type and form of exercise that is most suited for you, depending on your age and medical history. This will get you started on a systematic step-by-step approach. It also greatly reduces the risk of unwanted problems arising from exercise. I have heard people say that the exercise prescription given to them by their doctor was much simpler than the one they got from their spouse.

Elementary school children are required to have a physician's certificate before they enroll in any physical activities. You should, too. Why would you want to risk your spouse's, your children's, and your creditors' lives, all of whom are so dearly dependent on you, while you journey into a new adventure that requires a lifetime commitment? A stress EKG is an excellent test to take before starting on an exercise program, particularly if you are over 40 or in a high-risk group. (Those with a personal or family history of heart disease, high blood pressure, cholesterol, or long-term sedentary lifestyle are at high risk.)

When we exercise, our heart rate goes up to increase the amount of blood pumped to supply the extra oxygen needed by the exercising muscles. The blood pressure rises and the circulation to the skin increases to dissipate the excess heat by sweating. When you exercise regularly, the body adapts to stress by decreasing the heart rate response to exercise. This process is known as cardiac fitness or endurance. Over the long run, the heart develops collateral blood vessels to improve the circulation to the heart muscle. The skeletal muscles also adapt to exercise by using oxygen more efficiently. In addition, there is stimulation of the production of fat-burning enzymes with exercise.

To promote the production of fat-burning enzymes, you need to jump rope for 12 minutes, jog for 15 minutes, bicycle for 20 minutes, or walk briskly for 45 minutes. Twelve minutes of aerobics helps you to build, over months, a bigger fireplace that can burn many fat logs. The growth of fat-burning enzymes is the real purpose of exercising. You want more fat-burning enzymes so a year from now, your body will become a fat-burning machine instead of a fat-storing machine. The more muscles you use, the less time you need to spend exercising. When you start using the big muscles in the lower body, you will get a whole-body systemic effect.

There are many muscles in the upper body, but an upper-body exercise is not quite aerobic because the proportion of muscles used in comparison to total body weight is small. While exercising, if you can talk normally and are breathing deeply but comfortably, then you are almost certainly in the training zone.

Types of Exercises

There are three types of exercises:
- Stretching exercise
- Aerobic exercise
- Strength training exercise

Stretching Exercise

Stretching exercises are very important before getting involved in brisk aerobic activity. Stretching exercises help to relax your muscles and prevent any muscle spasms or cramps. Descriptions of different forms of stretching exercises can be found in books on sports medicine or running.

As you hold your hands up at shoulder level, push the palms of your hands against a wall and gently press for a couple of seconds. Wall-pushing activity helps you to stretch your arm muscles. Repeat this exercise three to four times, if you survive the first attempt. Then, touch the floor with the flat palms of your hands while standing, to stretch your belly and waist muscles. Repeat this exercise two to three times. Similarly, leg muscles can be stretched three to four times to relax them. You can stretch your neck muscles by turning your neck in different directions three to four times.

Aerobic Exercise

Aerobic exercise means a steady exercise, an exercise that demands an uninterrupted output from your muscles for a certain amount of time. The word aerobic means air, specifically, the oxygen in the air. The muscles need oxygen for their function, and their craving for oxygen goes up dramatically when they are exercised.

The longer you exercise, the more oxygen your muscles demand. This is partly due to an increase in heart rate. When muscles fail to get enough oxygen, they are forced to work under anaerobic conditions. During the anaerobic state, there is a build-up of lactic acid that causes lingering pains in those overworked sore muscles.

You can stimulate lipoprotein lipase, a fat-dissolving enzyme in your body, by doing any one of these activities:

- Jumping rope for 12 minutes
- Running for 15 minutes
- Bicycling for 20 minutes
- Walking continuously for 45 minutes

Two six-minute sessions are not equivalent to a twelve-minute exercise. Aerobic exercises performed daily can greatly help you to control your weight, especially when it is coupled with reduced calorie intake. The U.S. Department of Agriculture, in a 1993 report, affirmed that people who exercise moderately while dieting have much better weight-loss results.

Running: We generally consider running or jogging as synonymous with exercise. Undoubtedly, running is the most accepted, feasible, and practical form of aerobic exercise that you can make part of your daily life. The sustained, coordinated, and rhythmic actions involving large groups of muscles from areas such as the legs and the hips provide the most cardiovascular benefits. Running also enables us to take off or deduct a good number of calories from our fatty deposits. Good running shoes, along with cool comfortable clothes, can put you in the runner's lane in no time. Nowadays, several indoor facilities provide jogging tracks for your heart's delight. Or else you can create your own jogging trail around your breakfast table. Decorate your table with your favorite high fat, high calorie, and high taste foods. By the time you go around your dining table a couple of hundred times, your appetite would be so well served that you no longer feel like indulging in your familiar and festive eating habits. When you jog in the neighborhood, be sure to watch out for those tree branches reaching down in solitude to scalp your forehead. By all means, smell the roses and admire the people who provide you with such pleasant scenery. Who knows, your best friend may be living right next door to you, waiting for your humble friendship.

Bicycling: Bicycle riding provides similar cardiovascular benefits, provided you ride at a steady speed for at least 20 minutes. When you bicycle on the sidewalk, watch out for those tree trunks so that you don't return home with wooden dentures. Wet, slippery, and busted sidewalks can add an extra thrill to your riding skills. Whether you want to keep your head up or down while riding the bicycle depends on your confidence level. It also depends on how eagerly you want to avoid a head-on collision with another compulsive, aggressive, and impatient bicycle rider, or an elderly couple merely walking alongside. Your cardiovascular benefits are not directly proportional to the privileged price tag of your bicycle, but to the amount of time you spend riding that bicycle.

A stationary bicycle: It may solve the problem of risking your life on the main street. It also can eliminate your weather-related excuses. You can exercise on your stationary bicycle while watching TV, or while reading this information in ebook format. Your cardiovascular benefits are not directly proportional to the price tag of your bicycle, but to the amount of time you spend on it.

Jumping rope: This is what I call a solution to an excuse by an ever-running, ever-busy executive. If you are one of those fortunate individuals, or if you think you travel all the time, the jump rope could be your best exercise gear. You can use it right in your office, provided that you visit your office. When you travel, you can still complete your 12 minutes of exercise using a jump rope while rehearsing your business interviews in the tranquility of your mind in the hotel room.

Walking: Walking is better than sitting, sleeping, or doing nothing. Walking provides many benefits. You can walk anytime during the day or night. You don't need any special gear other than a pair of simple sneakers. When you are walking, you can have a nice conversation with your friend, listen to your favorite music, or window shop. You could also do bird watching, stargazing in the moonlight, or watch your own lingering shadow. People who walk for 45 minutes without interruption derive similar cardiovascular benefits to those who jog for 15 minutes or bicycle for 20 minutes.

If you are someone who for any medical reason can't run or jog, you may love to continue your exercise program by walking daily. I recommend that you choose a cooler climate and a place such as a park for your walks. If the weather is not ideal, you can walk in a large shopping mall where the climate is controlled. I would propose that you leave your purse or handbag in the car, before you enter the mall, so you will not be tempted to offset the benefits of your walking exercise by indulging in an ice cream party.

Target Heart Rate

The normal resting pulse rate for men is about 72 beats per minute, while for women it is 80 beats per minute. You should check your pulse several times during the day to get your average resting pulse rate. As your physical fitness improves, your resting pulse will come down. Very athletic individuals occasionally have a resting pulse as low as 35.

Here is a simple, easy-to-follow, easy-to-remember formula to determine your maximum heart rate for your age group:

Subtract your age from 220 to arrive at your ideal maximum heart rate.

Your target heart rate zone is 65% to 85% of your maximum heart rate. When you exercise, you want to maintain your heart rate in the target heart rate zone. The closer you are to the higher target heart rate, the more cardiovascular benefit you get. You don't get any additional cardiac benefit by going beyond your target zone. You may have to vary the duration and the intensity of your exercise to maintain your heart rate during your exercise session. If you stay in the training zone, a long, gentle workout is just as effective as a shorter, more intense workout.

The target heart rate zone applies to approximately 60 percent of the population. These people can make good use of pulse monitoring during and after exercise to judge the intensity of their exercise.

Certain medicines can alter heart rates, in some patients. Pulse rate as a measure of exercise intensity is not as reliable in this group. Others may have a high pulse rate to start with and an accelerated heart rate response to exercise. I have seen heart rate jump to 150 per minute in less than a minute in anxious people on a treadmill.

Obese people also do better with low-intensity activity when they first start an exercise program. Fit people burn fat well at higher intensities of exercise compared to overweight people. Emotional stress can be just as taxing as physical stress. Therefore, you can't judge your performance by the pulse rate or the target heart rate alone. Your overall well-being, coupled with your comfort during exercise, should be the determining factor. Remember that exercise is not an endpoint, but an interesting and essential step in the journey toward a Heart Healthy Lifestyle.

Caloric Expense Chart	
Activity and speed	Calories/hr
Jumping rope	750
Jogging at 5.5 mph	660
Jogging at 7.0 mph	920
Bicycle riding at 6 mph	240
Bicycle riding at 12 mph	410
Walking at 3 mph	320
Walking at 4.5 mph	440

Let's take a look at the calorie chart listed above. If you were to jog at a speed of 5.5 miles per hour, you would spend 660 calories in an hour. Thirty minutes of jogging per day results in the loss of 330 calories. If you cut down your calorie intake by 150 to 170 calories per day (the number in your favorite dessert), you will have a net loss of 500 calories per day or 3500 calories per week. Isn't it strange that each pound of fat has 3500 calories? Now you can see how the simple addition of numbers on a daily basis can mean a steady but definite weight reduction of one pound per week. Therefore, a combination of modest calorie reduction and regular exercise is the key to steady weight loss.

Pulse rate: You'll need a stopwatch or clock with a sweep-second hand. You can find your pulse on the outer side of your wrist. Sometimes it's difficult to find the pulse in the wrists of women and older people. You can locate the pulse in your neck. By putting your fingertips against the side of your neck, just below your jaw. Then, count your pulse for fifteen seconds, and multiply that by four to get the pulse rate.

Chapter 17

Exercise-Part 2
Exercise is the key to your wellness
Dine & Dance

Strength Training Exercise

If you think that exercise is hazardous to your health, you may be interested to know that you lose about half a pound of muscle mass each year. The calories that would otherwise have been burned by the lost muscle mass end up being stored as fat. I hate to be the one to point out that this is one of the causes of middle-age lower-body spread. If you consider the middle-age spread a threat to your graceful silhouette, then you can do something about it. The good news is that you can preserve your artistic presence by enrolling yourself in a combination of strength training exercises, aerobic exercises, and a low-fat diet. Exercise helps to trim your waist and broaden your smile.

Ladies, you need strength training exercises more than men do, not only to enhance your splendid elegance, but also to strengthen your tender bones along with the muscles, to reduce the risk of developing osteoporosis (thinning of the bones that signal the encroachment upon your youth by age).

While we are on the subject of age, I want to mention that strength training exercises also can benefit you in your golden years, which Erma Bombeck refers to as the Metallic Age. The metallic age is the twilight of life, heralded by silver hair, gold fillings, steel hips, and bronze spots, among others.

Henny Youngman said, "Even when you are pushing 70, you still need more exercise."

An elderly lady asked me, "Doc, do you think going back and forth in a swinging chair is a good exercise?"

I said, "Sure is . . . for the rocking chair."

Strength training exercises: They will enable you to improve your muscle strength, so you can share in the joy of tossing up your grandchildren and catching them as they come down, besides lifting your own groceries without herniating yourself to the ground. Strength training exercises don't take any more of your time than you would normally spend in inventing reasons not to enroll yourself in an exercise program. I recommend 2 to 5 pounds of weight for ladies, and 5 to 10 pounds of weight for men to strengthen their arm muscles.

Your strength training session should include a minimum of eight exercises involving the major muscles of your arms and legs. Perform each movement slowly and steadily for maximum benefit. Repeat each exercise 8 to 12 times for each group of muscles. Expect some muscle soreness for the first few days, but not sharp pain, especially in the joints. At the beginning of your training program, try to stretch your muscles without any weights. If you can't pass that stage, you had better consult your doctor.

Most of the aerobic exercises also help to strengthen your leg muscles. In addition, you can try lifting weights with your legs or working your thigh muscles against resistance. If you are a member of a health club, you can use various types of equipment to enable you to work your legs against resistance. If you can't afford a membership at a country club, and you can't spend a fortune to buy the required equipment, you can still achieve similar results with heel lifting, pushups, and stretching the thigh muscles. You can buy an exercise videotape and study the various exercises that strengthen different groups of muscles. If the exercise videotape starts collecting dust after several months in solitude, maybe it's a good idea to return it to the store, so other people waiting in line to surpass your early enthusiasm, may get a chance.

Avoid Exercise-Related Injuries

If you happen to be one of those genetic procrastinators who believe that nothing should be tried for the first time, then exercise injuries should not be the first item on your worry list. However, if you decide to come out of your warm, tranquil, and sedentary cocoon, and venture into the world of exercise, become fluent in body exercise. Here are some tips that could save many trips to emergency care centers.

1. Take time: Build your exercise program over several weeks to months, instead of cramming your course over a weekend. Besides, there is no point in ruining someone else's weekend, even though you could. Start your program at a very low level of exercise and gradually build your activity, allowing your muscles and joints to undergo natural adaptation to increased physical demand.

2. Listen to your body: If you pay attention to the signals coming from your joints, muscles, and limbs, you will be able to avoid any serious problems. There is a disparity between the bossy, pushy, and demanding thoughts radiating from your brain and the way your subordinate, unblemished, and unexplored muscles and joints respond to those signals, even though they are interconnected by one of the most highly evolved neural connections in existence. Don't try to whip your muscles when they cry in soreness and stiffness, or curl up in cramps. A simple persistent ache or soreness, misinterpreted by you as muscle spasm, could result in long-term disability. There is nothing worse in life than a disability that is not covered by Workers' Compensation. The symptoms that you experience may be a sign to slow down or totally eliminate a particular type of activity.

3. Overexertion: If you push beyond your physical limit, you may experience chest pain (stress pain), shortness of breath, or neck pain. These symptoms may also represent heart problems. Hence, let your activities be dictated more by your physical fitness and stamina than by some uncompromising numbers on a chart that were put together some 30 years ago by someone who can't even spell your first name. Dr. Charles W. Jarvis, a great humorous speaker from San

Marcos, Texas, said, "People have a lot of common sense, right? However, they haven't used any. It is sitting right there where God put it. Ladies (and gentlemen), what I am trying to say is, use that God-given common sense; it's cheap, it's yours, and it's good."

4. Out door tips: When you are exercising outdoors, don't blame the meteorologist. He can't order the weather specifically designed for your exercise regimen. Just stick your nose outside the door. If it turns red or blue, or feels numb, then you know you could use a warm jogging suit. Well, Christmas is right around the corner. So, just include a jogging suit wish, along with perhaps a jogging wish, in your list to Saint Nick. If you are lucky, you may see yourself running through next year's Christmas shopping in your jogging suit. While you are at it, you might as well shop for more jogging costumes and gear to match the other three seasons. After all, Dr. Jarvis says that you need to keep up with your neighbors, who are exercising regularly to keep up with you.

5. Foods: Many food conflicts with your exercise program, in more ways than one. If you eat too much, then you don't feel like exercising. If you don't exercise, you feel as though you are giving your body excess weight by just living and breathing. Then you have to eat more to support those excess living cells. The best way to end the cycle of misery is to exercise vigorously for 20 to 30 minutes, and settle down for your scrumptious meal. If you don't eat more than your share, you don't need to sweat too much.

6. Environmental factors: They can add a special touch to your jogging thrills. Hard cement surfaces are more likely to injure your feet than a level grass field or a dirt path. Special jogging shoes may protect you from some of those injuries. But don't expect the protection to match the price tag of your jogging shoes. Use other protective gear such as goggles when required; land on your heels, rather than on the ball of your feet or your knees, when you are jogging. Please remember that traffic signs were created by the people, for the people, including the street joggers. If you are an avid bicycle rider, kindly extend courtesy to your fellow bicycle riders, so they don't have to go out of the way to send you to the hospital. A head-on crash by two or more bicycle riders, though rare, can be dangerous.

It's not against the bicycle religion to lift your head occasionally, especially when your own life is riding on those fast-moving, slender wheels. If you must invade the streets on your bike, please ride in the direction of the traffic. Better yet, stand on the sidewalk and watch for the signal radiating from the automobile drivers to their bicycle counterparts to appreciate the wisdom of those drivers.

A Typical Exercise Session

Warm-up. Dedicate 5 minutes of your life to each warm-up session. Begin with stretching your arm and leg muscles. Then, stretch your back and abdominal muscles. Finally, stretch your neck muscles. These stretching exercises enable your muscles to stretch before they are put to more vigorous use, thus preventing any undue strain on the muscles or the ligaments when they are involved in vigorous rhythmic action during an exercise session.

Exercise: Before jogging, first try walking and then switch to brisk walking. If you have trouble walking, you may consider at least getting up from your bed. Remember that one small step could start you on a lifelong adventure. The aerobic exercise part of the program should include a sustained brisk activity such as jogging, running, walking, or bicycling. When you are exercising, make sure your heart rate stays in the target heart rate zone of 60 to 85 percent of your maximum heart rate. Continue your exercise for at least 15 to 30 minutes. Avoid any distractions such as the squeaking noise coming from the refrigerator door or the messages flashing on your TV channel.

Cool-down: Entering a cool-down period doesn't necessarily mean that you should immediately immerse yourself in a tank of cold water. During this phase, gradually decrease your level of activity, but continue to walk. This allows your body to relax gradually. Abrupt stopping can cause dizziness and weakness due to pooling of blood in the lower part of your body, especially when the pumping action of the leg muscles comes to a sudden halt after working for several minutes. Repeat your stretching exercises to loosen up your muscles before you stop your exercise session. When you exercise, your heart rate typically reaches a maximum for your age, and it will not beat any faster, no matter how much harder you exercise.

When you start a new exercise, you may have to stop several times to check your pulse until you know exactly how hard to exercise to reach the target heart rate. Many people find that after several weeks of training, their hearts don't reach the training zone at the same level of exercise. This simply means that in most cases you should run faster, pedal with more resistance, or jump higher. If this doesn't appeal to you, simply switch to a different type of exercise to get your heart into its target zone.

If you are terribly out of shape, even brisk walking may put you out of breath. Then, you should decrease the intensity of your exercise, not the duration of exercise. One man said that when he first started, he had trouble just rolling in his bed, but he made it.

The Key to Your Successful Exercise Program

The key to a successful exercise program begins with your determination. Only you can make this important lifetime decision.

Let me emphasize again that you are the one who is going to benefit from your exercise program. In these chapters on exercise, I have described the type of exercise, duration of exercise, location, and the equipment necessary to help you with your exercise program. Some people prefer to exercise in the early morning hours, while others find it most suitable during the late evening hours. I also have seen people using their lunch breaks for exercise activities. How much time you are willing to spend on your exercise program depends on your goals. If you want to stay in shape, build your muscles, and enhance your silhouette, you need at least 30 minutes of exercise, three to four times a week. If you plan to lose weight, you may want to exercise more often and for longer durations. Again, it doesn't mean that you have to work harder or push yourself beyond your target heart rate zone.

Begin your exercise with the least amount of stress, then gradually build up as your strength and stamina improve. I want to stress again that you need a lifetime commitment. We are talking about lifestyle changes for good, are we not?

Your exercise program doesn't have to be restricted to 30 minutes, three times a week. Throughout the day, you can perform certain activities that can greatly enhance your muscle strength and help you to spend calories.

You can use stairs instead of the elevators when you are going up or down a couple of flights. You may try to park your car at the end of the parking lot, rather than going around in circles for ten minutes looking for an open spot in the front row. The front row is reserved for those who can't walk. As you walk through the parking lot, you not only can spend some calories, but also look for the model of your next dream car.

Try replacing your coffee breaks with simple exercise breaks. Instead of watching television or listening to music at home in seclusion, you can use your iPod, iPhone, or iPad and complete a 30 minute walk while listening to your favorite music or reading your favorite eBooks, such as Heart Healthy Living and others.

If you want to go to your neighborhood grocery store that is less than a mile away, you might consider using your bike instead of driving your car. Make sure there is no hurricane in the forecast for the next 2 hours before you start. Guess what? You can kill two birds with one stone—exercise and shopping.

Practice deep abdominal muscle exercises whenever you can find a couple of free minutes. When time permits, practice lifting your heels up, which can strengthen your muscles.

Notes:

Chapter 18

Weight Control

Houston, we've got a problem!

Are You Serious About Losing Weight?

Recently, my hometown Houston was crowned, for the second time, with the exemplary title "The fattest city in America." Houston! we've got a problem!

It is not just Houston. Approximately two out of every three adults in America are overweight. As the baby boomers enter their late fifties and sixties, they need to consider the adverse effects of obesity on their cardiovascular system.

Some time ago, Jack, a young, tall, oversized Texan, came to my office for a checkup. As I was taking his medical history, he exclaimed, "Doc, you have been sizing me over like I'm pregnant with octuplets! I know what you are going to ask me next."

"And that is?" I queried.

"If I have been on a diet program before? Or, maybe, if I have considered bariatric surgery in the past?" he replied, with a penetrating look into my eyes.

"Have you?" I smiled.

"Let me tell you, Dr. Nik! I have been on twenty diet programs in the past 20 years. I must have lost 1000 pounds and gained back 1000 pounds. The last thing I want to hear from you is that I need another diet program."

"What did you do between your diet programs, may I ask?"

"I ate the usual—steak, cheeseburgers, fries, ice cream, and chips. Anything else you would like to know?" He chuckled.

"Jack, the trouble with you is that you are not consistent. You gain weight, lose weight, and then again, gain weight and lose weight. We in the medical profession call that the rhythm method of girth control!"

"Is it supposed to be funny?" He looked puzzled.

"Yes. You do not need another short-term diet plan. I can agree with you one hundred percent."

"What do you mean?"

"What you do need is a well-balanced, Heart Healthy Lifestyle, designed especially for you," I replied.

"There you go—as I suspected, another diet plan!" He sighed.

"This is not a diet plan. It is about re-engineering your lifestyle. It is about helping you understand what is at stake and how you can take control of your destiny. It is about achieving a balanced lifestyle," I said.

"Dr. Nik, I just came here for some blood pressure pills."

"What about your cholesterol level?"

"It's high, that's all I know," he said.

"And your blood sugar level?"

"Borderline."

"Any chest pain?"

"Yes, and no. I did not have any when I came. Now, I am feeling some answering your interrogation."

"Shortness of breath?"

"Only when I walk to the refrigerator during a football game." He chuckled.

"Arthritis?"

"A little!"

"What does that mean?"

"My back hurts when I exert myself."

"Did anyone tell you that most of your symptoms may be related to one thing—your weight?" I asked.

"There you go again! Rub it in, Dr. Nik, rub it in!" he growled as he rubbed his fist backwards and forwards on the table.

"What is your height?" I continued.

"Five feet, seven inches."

"Your weight?"

"302 pounds, give or take 20 pounds."

"Belt size?"

"Now you are getting on my nerves," he replied, galled.

"What if I fixed all your problems with one thing?" I challenged.

"You've got a pill! What's the name of the pill, Dr. Nik? How do you spell it?" He asked, excited.

"*L-o-s-e W-e-i-g-h-t!*" I dramatized.

"I'm out of here!" he stood up.

"Go ahead. I will even skip your charges for this visit."

"Dr. Nik, let me ask you a question. Have you ever been on any diet program yourself?" he asked, and looked at the door.

"I hate diet programs, I hate liquid protein, and I hate diet pills."

"Then how can you recommend one for others?"

"This is a *lifestyle*—a long-term, life-transforming journey."

"What does that mean in English?"

"It means that as you try to lose weight, you pay attention to reducing risks associated with being overweight, such as high cholesterol, blood pressure, and elevated blood sugar levels. You must replace your unhealthy eating patterns with healthy habits, by following the principles outlined in my book."

"Can I have a cheeseburger with bacon and fries?"

"Not quite!"

"So, you mean to tell me that you are convinced that all my symptoms are related to my extra weight?" he asked.

"That's right," I affirmed.

"Well, no doctor has ever explained to me before that overweight could lead to so many problems!" he said, returning to his seat. "What contributes to excess weight—bones, fat, or muscles?"

"Most extra weight results from the accumulation of excess fat around the belt and buns."

"Aren't you getting a little personal here?" he said. "Why is it only fat? Why not muscle?"

"Good question," I said. "Any excess food energy that is not immediately used is converted into fat. The body can store a very limited amount of carbohydrates (400 to 500 g) as glycogen, very little protein, and yet an unlimited quantity of fat—in all the wrong places!"

"So, how do I prevent fat buildup?"

"First, you should cut down your calories."

"What is the minimum calorie count you recommend per day?"

"I recommend no less than 1200 calories per day."

"How did you come up with a minimum of 1200 calories?" he asked.

"People who eat less than 1200 calories per day go into a catabolic state, where their bodies begin to break down muscle protein to sustain life. That is why people who are on a starvation diet or a very low-calorie diet look weak, emaciated, and sick. And, of course, that is not good for their health," I stressed.

"You said 1200 calories, but of what—carbs, proteins, or fat?" he asked.

"That is an excellent question. We use 1200 calorie feedings for patients whoa are unable to eat, in the hospitals. It is a well-balanced diet with the right amount of carbs (30%), proteins (30%), and fats (30%). What type of diet programs have you tried in the past?"

"I have tried diets recommending everything from low carbs to high proteins. I have even tried high-fat diets. You name it, I've tried it!"

"Did any of those diets work?"

"For a little while."

"Then what happened?"

"You know, you really can't live on just low carbs, liquid proteins, or bacon and sausage for very long. Definitely not for a lifetime!"

"You just made my point. You stole my words. Now, we are on the same page." I smiled.

"What do you mean?"

"You correctly pointed out the inherent problem with most diet programs. They are an artificial lifestyle that lasts only as long as your overzealous obsession with their program persists. Once the honeymoon period is over, you are back to your old habits, right?" I probed. "You see, there is no one diet plan that covers all aspects of life."

"Then what is the secret of your weight control program?"

"I follow two vital principles based on sound scientific evidence. First, in order to see any weight reduction, you must reduce your total calorie intake. Eating double, jumbo, or extra servings of any one food, no matter how healthy, is not going to reduce your weight."

"What will calorie reduction do for me?"

"It will prevent your body from further accumulation of fat."

"But I want to get rid of the excess fat I already have."

"That brings us to the second vital principle of my weight control philosophy."

"What is that?"

"Exercise, exercise, and more steady exercise!"

"What happens when I exercise?"

"When you exercise, your body depletes its carbohydrate energy sources (glycogen). Next, your body begins to burn excess fat for energy. The body also adapts by producing more fat burning enzyme called lipoprotein lipase, that burns more fat for energy."

"Will any form of exercise work?"

"Short bursts of exercise will generally burn only carbohydrate reserves stored as glycogen, not fat."

"So how can I burn fat?"

"You have to engage yourself in exercises of moderate intensity for a long duration. These exercises will primarily burn fat for their constant energy needs."

"That's interesting. What moderate intensity, long duration exercise do you suggest?" He leaned back.

"A one-hour brisk walk will burn 150 calories."

"That's it?" Jack exclaimed, disappointed.

"Yep, it is not even the number of calories in a soft drink."

"That's unfair," he said, wiping the sweat off his forehead with his index finger.

"I am sorry, my friend. Would you like a Kleenex?"

"No, I'll just use the *Nikam's Diet* handout you gave me." He chuckled.

"But moving on, now we come back to my first point—calorie reduction."

"That stuff again?"

"You must reduce the intake of unnecessary calories so you won't have to struggle later to burn those empty calories."

"That makes sense. But how do I put it into practice?"

"Before you embark on *Nikam's Diet* instructions, you need to have a complete medical checkup, including blood tests evaluating your electrolytes, liver, and kidney functions. Then ascertain your actual height and weight and take an inventory of your vital statistics. If you are over forty, an exercise test would be advisable."

"Then what?"

"While you are taking the inventory, make sure to take two pictures of yourself, one from the front view and one from the side."

"Why, I'm not a prisoner?" he inquired.

"Well, in a way you are a prisoner. You are a prisoner of your own weight. While taking the picture, make sure you hold a card that reads *KHAIDI: 01-01-05*. Post a copy of the picture on the refrigerator and place another copy next to your bed."

"Khaidi? What does that mean?"

"It means *prisoner* in the Indian language."

"Are you serious?"

"You bet!"

"What does the number represent? Is that my prison ID?" he joked.

"The number represents the date the picture was taken. It allows you to compare your future progress or regress. When you take another picture a couple of months later, it will inspire you to change your plans or select a new doctor," I smiled.

"Clever! I may take you up on that idea."

Unmoved by his response, I continued, "Did you say your weight was 302 pounds?"

"Yeah . . . what about it?"

"Okay; now, let's figure out your BMI," I said.

"Wait a minute! What is BMI?"

"BMI stands for body mass index. It determines how much surplus fat you have."

"What is a normal BMI?"

"The normal BMI range is between 19 and 24.9."

"What is my BMI?"

"Your BMI is 31.3."

"Uh-oh! Is that dangerously high?"

"It is well above the normal limit. Our aim is to get your BMI close to 25, which is the upper limit of normal."

"How do I do that?"

"In order to get your BMI to 25, you will have to reduce your weight from 302 to 180 pounds."

"120 pounds of what? What part of me?"

"That is an excellent question. I am talking about getting rid of 120 pounds of your fat, not muscle or brain tissue."

"How did you conclude that I have brain tissue to spare?"

"No comment," I said.

"Back to the main point!"

"Okay, okay! Let me explain what 120 pounds of fat mean. Basically, it is stored energy. Each gram of fat has nine calories, and each pound of fat has 400 grams or 3600 calories (400 g x 9 = 3600). Now, let as agree that you want to lose 40 pounds in your first phase of this new lifestyle. To get rid of 40 pounds of fat, you just have to burn 144,000 calories! How about that?"

"God have mercy! Let me see if I understand you correctly. You said that I can lose 150 calories by walking for an hour. That means, if I walk for 1000 hours, I should be able to lose 40 pounds, right? Dr. Nik, I don't have 1000 hours. I work 14 hour days. I have business meetings, dinner meetings. . . you get the picture. How about a pill?"

"Well, it looks like a lot of calories until you break it down."

"I hope so. You lost me there for second." He looked disinterested.

Observing the lack of interest in his eyes, I said, "You need a realistic goal or a vision. Let us assume that you want to achieve that

40 pound weight loss goal in one year. Since there are 365 days in a year, walking 2.63 hours daily would enable you to lose 40 pounds without ever changing your diet habits."

"But, Doc, I can't walk 2.63 hours each day. That's 365 days without a break?"

"Good, now you are thinking!" I said.

"Do you have a plan B?"

"I realize that most people do not have an extra 2.63 hours each day to walk. Of course, I have a plan B and even a plan C. My plan B calls for a 400-calorie reduction from your present diet if you cannot burn those calories each day by walking."

"Okay, from what meal do I reduce 400 calories?" he asked.

"Do you like pecan pie?"

"I love it. But my wife has set a limit of two or three servings per week."

"If it was up to you?"

"I would eat it for lunch and dinner." He smiled.

"Do you know how many calories there are in a single piece of pecan pie?"

"Doc! Do you think I worry about calories when I am enjoying my favorite pecan pie?"

"You mean when you are stuffing your fat cells?" I quipped.

"Okay. How many calories?"

"400 calories!"

"You are not going to take away my dessert, are you?"

"No, I'm trying to help you understand how to get rid of those forty pounds of excess fat.

"If you give up your dessert, then you are reducing your average daily intake of calories by one hundred and seventy one (400 x 3 = 1200 calories per week or 1200/7 = 170 calories per day). Now, you only have to walk 1.5 hours a day to burn the remaining 230 calories."

"Still, Doc, I don't have an extra 1.5 hours per day."

"Can you walk for an hour a day?" I asked.

"Maybe," Jack sighed.

"In that case, you are burning 150 calories per day with this newly discovered Heart Healthy Lifestyle, by walking for an hour each day. Then, if you reduce your calorie intake by 250 to 300 calories per day, you are within striking distance of realizing your target weight at the end of one year."

"What if I want to achieve the same results in six months?"

"Then you will have to double your efforts. That means you have to achieve a 800 calorie negative balance from your present level."

"Is it possible?"

"Let's look at it more closely. You burn only 150 calories with your exercise. The remaining calories have to be counted in terms of reduced intake. That means you have to reduce your calorie intake by almost 600 to 650 calories per day."

"Doc, I'm not eating that much to begin with."

"You are eating something, aren't you?"

"I don't know how much or how many calories. How do I find out?"

"That's why I designed a special chart to help you balance your calories."

"How is that going to help me?"

"There, you write down what you eat for breakfast, lunch, and dinner. Make sure that you include your snacks and drinks, even though you don't count those as food."

"Then what do I do?"

"Then, you look at the Heart Healthy calorie chart provided on my website. This chart serves two purposes. First, it lets you know if the food you are eating is heart healthy. If it is not on the chart then it may not be."

"What about prime rib, is it heart healthy?"

"I'm sorry, Bud, too much saturated fat."

"Ice cream?"

"Well, there is no need to scream! Second, the purpose of the chart is to provide you with the approximate calories, carbs, proteins, fat, fiber, and cholesterol for each food item. Write these figures down and at the end of the day add them up. Make sure to subtract the number of calories that you burned during exercise."

"Doc, do I have to do this all my life?"

"Did you learn phonics in school? Are you using phonics in your conversation?"

"Yes."

"Do you think about them every time you utter a word?"

"No, but what are you getting at?"

"Well, just as phonics became second nature to you, so will a Heart Healthy Lifestyle. As you track your eating habits for two to three weeks, you will learn your nutritional phonics. The next time you see an unhealthy food, those numbers will be dancing in front of your eyes as you to grab the wrong food while cruising through the cafeteria line."

"I didn't know you were a shrink!"

"I'm trying to help you shrink your fat mass."

"Are you playing on my mind? Is this some kind of a . . ."

"Psychotherapy, you mean?"

"Yeah! That is the word I was looking for."

"Okay Jack, now you see a pecan pie—what should immediately come to your mind?"

"Pecan pie, 400 calories, a second on my lips and the rest of the time on my hips. Run, run, run, Brother Jack."

"You are a fast learner! Common sense, Jack. That's what I'm trying to cultivate among people. Now, let me ask you a question: What kind of work do you do?"

"I'm a software engineer."

"So you softly wear your rear on the office chair for 8 to 10 hours a day, right?"

"I hope my boss doesn't know that."

"Approximately how many calories do you consume per day?"

"Maybe around 2000 calories," he said.

"If you have not been able to lose weight on a 2000 calorie diet, you can systematically reduce your Take calorie intake down to 1200 calories per day, without compromising a Heart Healthy Lifestyle," I emphasized.

"That's it! I got it. If I cut my daily calorie intake by 800, I do not even have to exercise. What do you think, Doc?"

"That's right. You don't even need to see me any more, 'cause I know you are not getting anywhere."

"I knew that you had something up your sleeve to spoil my plot."

"Remember, I said that there are two basic principles in weight control."

"I don't remember."

"Then let me repeat it again. First, you restrict your calorie intake to prevent any further fat buildup. Second, you engage in a regular exercise program to burn off excess fat in your body."

"Is exercise the only way to get rid of fat from my body? How about a fat burning pill, Dr. Nik? Why haven't you come up with a fat burning pill? You could be making a killing with that pill."

"There are already a bunch of diet pills claiming to be fat burners. If you belong and firmly believe in a popular pill-popping culture, you have come to the wrong place, Jack. Here, we are concerned not only about your weight today and tomorrow, but also about your heart and overall health, quality of life, and longevity. We practice medicine the old-fashioned way. We encourage people to sweat it out—if it is good for weight control, it should be good for your heart.

"Okay. You don't have to massage it so deep."

"Study your daily calorie intake and expense (you know how to balance your checkbook, don't you?"

"My wife takes care of that. Remember, you said let your wife handle the money."

"Day by day, trim your Take calories, increase intake of heart healthy choices, and you will gradually notice your pants getting loose. Then, you may feel a sense of exhilaration running through your body."

"I can't wait! Now, coming back to the diet part, which religion do you belong to: carbs, proteins, or fats?"

"My religion is cardiology, my culture is long-term Heart Healthy Lifestyle. These are the reasons why my program goes well beyond just short-term weight control. I am also interested in preserving your heart, improving your quality of life, increasing your longevity, while you enjoy normal foods without being addicted to diet pills, carbs, or whatever has not worked in the past. I teach you what are essential proteins, essential fatty acids, vitamins, fiber, and water; and why they are important to your overall well-being.

"What's wrong with carbs?"

"Carbs are fine when used in moderation. Let me dispel the myths and misunderstandings about restricting carbs. General reduction in calories including carbs helps in maintaining an ideal body weight. I have also compiled a low glycemic carbs chart. When you are on a low-carb diet, make sure that you do not load your system with fats or proteins. This is one of the problems I have with the Atkins diet."

"What about low-fat diets?"

"Dean Ornish is a great proponent of low-fat diets. They are good. But, we need to understand the difference between what is ideal and what is practical. It would be ideal to reduce your fat intake to less than ten percent of the calories. However, it is practically impossible to reduce the fats to that level lifelong. Also, we have to realize that low-fat studies were done when we did not have powerful cholesterol lowering drugs or new forms of fat that are not absorbed. Now, we also have fats such as Benecol and Take Control that actually lower cholesterol levels. Besides, low-fat diets are not the best option for weight control. They are useful in reducing cholesterol and triglyceride levels."

He kept going. "What about high protein diets?"

"I feel moving from one food group to another may seem attractive and may serve as a selling point for certain diet programs, but eventually all macronutrients (large food components such as carbs, proteins and fats) provide energy besides providing essential cellular functions. You need a comprehensive lifestyle plan and a sound scientific concept behind such plan."

"Is too much protein bad?" he asked.

"Yes indeed. If you just eat protein all day long, you are going to get some serious health problems."

"I see you don't recommend any pills for weight control."

"I don't know of anyone who would willingly take diet pills all their life. I do know people eat the same kind of foods they grew up with for the most of their lives. However, helping people to maintain their weight, while letting them eat their own food is our mission and philosophy."

"Do I need follow-ups?" He looked worried about his fees.

"Most definitely. First, I need to determine if you are making progress or regress. Second, we can check your blood chemistries to make sure that your electrolytes are not out of control. I have seen several patients who had been on weight control pills coming to the emergency room with low electrolyte levels and I have even seen people who had cardiac arrhythmias. People who have been on a high-protein diet have also been shown to have low calcium and phosphate in the blood. Next, we will review your dietary charts to see how well you have been able to cheat. Finally, we can advise you on which items are best suited for your lifestyle in the long run."

"Why do people lose weight quickly initially?"

"When people lose weight, the initial three to five pounds of weight loss happens quickly. As you deplete the glycogen stores, your body gets rid of additional salt and water. Hence, you notice a quick three to five pound weight loss. However, losing fat mass takes time and a very strict regimen of calorie restriction combined with regular exercise."

"How much weight loss is ideal?"

"I would recommend a two pound weight loss per week. That will give you time to burn calories, restrict food intake, and allow your body to mobilize the fat in an orderly manner."

"What about the stretch marks?"

"If you lose weight on a steady basis and engage in aerobic and strengthening exercises, the skin will shrink over time. So your body becomes more compact and firm."

"Do all patients behave similarly?"

"Each person behaves uniquely in his or her own way toward weight control. Some people respond easily, while others have to struggle to get rid of one inch of waistline. There are many genetic and social components that need reprogramming."

"Why do some people have trouble losing weight?"

"The human body is the greatest chemical factory ever created on the face of this earth. If you add to that the genetic factors about which we know very little, and individual personalities, we have too many variables which are hard to control and cannot predict the outcome. Unfortunately, it is not always black and white. I learned this a long time ago dealing with cardiac surgery patients. When two patients with similar age and degree of heart disease went for heart surgery, their outcomes were quite different. It is not a mathematical equation, where two plus two equals four, or a business equation where one plus one equals three, the results are variable and only those who try will find out. Also note that only those people who try are the ones who are going to make a mistake. It is better to try and make a mistake than to live in misery all your life."

"What happens when I reach the target weight goal?"

"The best thing about this Heart Healthy Lifestyle program is that you don't have to change your diet very much. Since you are eating normal food selections and the right heart healthy foods, you continue to enjoy the same recipes and menus. You may have to reduce your extra calorie expense to some degree or increase your calorie intake if you are spending too many calories. Check with your talking scale and watch for your belt size and beltline. Your belt would immediately signal if you are headed in the wrong direction, so your belt and pants are your best perimeters!"

"What happens if my pants get a little tight?"

"It means your Heart Healthy Lifestyle is falling through the cracks. Do not feel bad; I have been there myself a few times. After all, we are human. We feel good for a while and then we get sidetracked and give up all the good things that we were doing to keep us on the right track. Then we need to go back to the drawing board and start at the zero point to see what things we were not doing right. Then we start all over again by rectifying the mistakes and trying to get back on track. Once again, after all, we are human. However, being constantly aware of the Heart Healthy Lifestyle every minute of our lives makes corrections of our mistakes a little bit easier."

"What is the relationship between weight and metabolism?

When you lose weight, your metabolism slows down, but if you maintain the same calorie intake, then you won't lose any more weight. In order to continue to lose weight, you should increase your metabolic needs by increasing your aerobic activities that burn more and more calories. That is one of the reasons that people lose weight for a while and stabilize and don't see much change. By building your muscles, you increase your muscle mass, which burns more calories in an efficient matter. So you can eat more and lose fat at the same time.

Determine How Much Weight You Need to Lose
Body Mass Index Table

BMI	19	20	21	22	23	24	25	26	27	28	29	30	31	32	33	34
Ht							Body Weight (pounds)									
58	91	96	100	105	110	115	119	124	129	134	138	143	148	153	158	162
59	94	99	104	109	114	119	124	128	133	138	143	148	153	158	163	168
60	97	102	107	112	118	123	128	133	138	143	148	153	158	163	168	174
61	100	106	111	116	122	127	132	137	143	148	153	158	164	169	174	180
62	104	109	115	120	126	131	136	142	147	153	158	164	169	175	180	186
63	107	113	118	124	130	135	141	146	152	158	163	169	175	180	186	191
64	110	116	122	128	134	140	145	151	157	163	169	174	180	186	192	197
65	114	120	126	132	138	144	150	156	162	168	174	180	186	192	198	204
66	118	124	130	136	142	148	155	161	167	173	179	186	192	198	204	210
67	121	127	134	140	146	153	159	166	172	178	185	191	198	204	211	217
68	125	131	138	144	151	158	164	171	177	184	190	197	203	210	216	223
69	128	135	142	149	155	162	169	176	182	189	196	203	209	216	223	230
70	132	139	146	153	160	167	174	181	188	195	202	209	216	222	229	236
71	136	143	150	157	165	172	179	186	193	200	208	215	222	229	236	243
72	140	147	154	162	169	177	184	191	199	206	213	221	228	235	242	250
73	144	151	159	166	174	182	189	197	204	212	219	227	235	242	250	257
74	148	155	163	171	179	186	194	202	210	218	225	233	241	249	256	264
75	152	160	168	176	184	192	200	208	216	224	232	240	248	256	264	272
76	156	164	172	180	189	197	205	213	221	230	238	246	254	263	271	279

Source: NIH

Heart Healthy Lifestyle

Nikam's Diet: Calorie Diet Sheet

Foods	Cal	Protein	Carb	Fats	Fiber	Chol
	1200	300 cal	400 cal	400 cal	>30 g	<300 mg
Breakfast						
1.						
2.						
3.						
4.						
5.						
Lunch						
1.						
2.						
3.						
4.						
5.						
Dinner						
1.						
2.						
3.						
4.						
5.						
Snacks						
1.						
2.						
3.						
Total Calorie Intake						
Exercise						
1						
2.						
Total Calorie Expense						

Nikam's Diet: 1200 Calorie Diet Sheet

Foods	% Cal	Cal	QNT	Food Sources
Proteins	30%	360	90.0 g	8 oz. of lean meat, grilled chicken, turkey. Eat fish >2 times a week. Kidney beans, chickpeas, whole wheat, peas, nuts <1 oz.
Fats, SFA	10%	120	13.3 g	In meats, dressings. Avoid coconut, butter.
Fats, USFA	20%	240	26.6 g	Canola oil, olive oil, avocado.
Carbs	30%	360	90.0 g	Whole wheat, fruits, All-Bran or Fiber One cereal. Avoid high glycemic index foods: sugar, white flour.
Fiber	5%	60	30-40 g	Metamucil (psyllium), high-fiber whole-wheat tortillas, All-Bran, Fiber One.
Alcohol	5%	60		If you desire, drink 5 oz. of red wine or one shot of hard liquor or a light beer.
Water			2-3 L	Most important part of the diet.
Salads			1	Lots of vegetables. Watch for croutons and fruit's sugar content.
Dressings				Use a fraction of the dressing.
Salt			2-4 g	Try lime-pepper. Avoid canned foods.
Vitamins/minerals A-Z			1	Helps to replenish all vitamins and minerals.
Diet soft drinks			OK	Watch for caffeine and salt.
Sugar substitutes			OK	Avoid pure sugar that has very high glycemic index.
Snacks				All-Bran or Fiber One cereal. 1 oz. chips has 150 calories and 8-10 g of fat; the rest is carbohydrates. Make your own fiber- and protein-rich baked spicy snacks.
Exercise		-300		30 min. walking, 20 min. biking, 15 min. jogging or 12 min. jumping rope will expend 150 calories. All other activities can more than make up the other 150 calories.

Nikam's Diet: 1500 Calorie Diet sheet

Foods	% Cal	Cal	QNT	Food Sources
Proteins	30%	450	113 g	8 oz. of lean meat, grilled chicken, turkey. Eat fish >2 times a week. Kidney beans, chickpeas, whole wheat, peas, nuts <1 oz.
Fats, SFA	10%	150	16.6 g	In meats, dressings. Avoid coconut, butter.
Fats, USFA	20%	300	33.3 g	Canola oil, olive oil, avocado.
Carbohydrates	30%	450	113 g	Whole wheat, fruits, All-Bran or Fiber One cereal. Avoid high glycemic index food: sugar, white flour.
Fiber	5%	75	30-40 g	Metamucil (psyllium), high-fiber whole-wheat tortillas, All-Bran, Fiber One.
Alcohol	5%	75		If you desire, take 5 oz. of red wine or one shot of hard liquor or a light beer.
Water			2-3 L	Most important part of the diet.
Salads			1	Lots of vegetables. Watch for croutons and fruit's sugar content.
Dressings				Use a fraction of the dressing.
Salt			2-4 g	Try lime-pepper. Avoid canned foods.
Vitamins/minerals A-Z			1	Helps to replenish all vitamins and minerals.
Diet soft drinks			OK	Watch for caffeine and salt.
Sugar substitutes			OK	Avoid pure sugar that has very high glycemic index
Snacks				All-Bran or Fiber One cereal. 1 oz. chips has 150 calories and 8-10 g of fat; the rest is carbohydrates. Make your own fiber- and protein-rich baked spicy snacks.
Exercise		-300		30 min. walking, 20 min. biking, 15 min. jogging or 12 min. jumping rope will expend 150 calories. All other activities can more than make up the other 150 calories.

Nikam's Diet: 1800 Calorie Diet Sheet

Foods	% Cal	Cal	QNT	Food Sources
Proteins	30%	360	90.0 g	8 oz. of lean meat, grilled chicken, turkey. Eat fish >2 times a week. Kidney beans, chickpeas, whole wheat, peas, nuts <1 oz.
Fats, SFA	10%	120	13.3 g	In meats, dressings. Avoid coconut, butter.
Fats, USFA	20%	240	26.6 g	Canola oil, olive oil, avocado.
Carbs	30%	360	90.0 g	Whole wheat, fruits, All-Bran or Fiber One cereal. Avoid high glycemic index foods: sugar, white flour.
Fiber	5%	60	30-40 g	Metamucil (psyllium), high-fiber whole-wheat tortillas, All-Bran, Fiber One.
Alcohol	5%	60		If you desire, drink 5 oz. of red wine or one shot of hard liquor or a light beer.
Water			2-3 L	Most important part of the diet.
Salads			1	Lots of vegetables. Watch for croutons and fruit's sugar content.
Dressings				Use a fraction of the dressing.
Salt			2-4 g	Try lime-pepper. Avoid canned foods.
Vitamins/minerals A-Z			1	Helps to replenish all vitamins and minerals
Diet soft drinks			OK	Watch for caffeine and salt.
Sugar substitutes			OK	Avoid pure sugar that has very high glycemic index.
Snacks				All-Bran or Fiber One cereal. 1 oz. chips has 150 calories and 8-10 g of fat; the rest is carbohydrates. Make your own fiber- and protein-rich baked spicy snacks.
Exercise		-300		30 min. walking, 20 min. biking, 15 min. jogging or 12 min. jumping rope will expend 150 calories. All other activities can more than make up the other 150 calories.

Chapter 19

Heart Attack & Sudden Death
Life is like a candle in the middle of a desert

Heart Attack

When someone feels some chest discomfort, the first reaction may be that it is related to gas or something that person ate. It may also signal a heart attack.

When someone is actually having a heart attack, time is of the essence. Every minute you delay in getting the necessary medical help, there is ongoing damage to the heart muscle. The longer a person waits, the more damage there is to the heart muscle. The extent of heart muscle damage that you sustain during a heart attack determines your survival chances and resulting development of heart failure.

Among the people who develop heart attacks, 40% to 50% of them do not make it to the hospital. They die either from severe heart muscle damage or fatal heart rhythm irregularities. Among those who make it to the hospital, another 7% to 9% die in the hospital from complications related to the heart attack.

How can we minimize heart muscle damage, save lives, and improve quality of life following a heart attack? This involves a team approach from the public, the emergency medical service, the hospitals, and the physicians involved in taking care of heart attack patients. Education, training, expedience, and appropriate application treatment options, such as blood thinners, emergency cardiac catheterization, and opening of the arterial blockages, can reduce disability and death following a heart attack.

What causes heart attacks? Heart attack results from a total blockage of a blood vessel supplying a region of a heart muscle. Initially, there is buildup of an atherosclerotic plaque (hardening of the arteries) that develops over decades. The final 5% to 10% of the final blockage results from development of a clot because of slowing of circulation in that region due to the severe obstruction. When this total blockage goes untreated, there is irreversible damage to the heart muscle which is eventfully replaced by scar tissue (assuming that you survive the initial threat and seek timely medical help).

What is the urgency? As I mentioned at the beginning, it is of paramount importance to unclog the artery to restore blood circulation with the hope of minimizing the heart muscle damage and improving survival. If we can unclog the artery within 60 to 90 minutes after the onset of a heart attack, we can reduce the in-hospital death rate from 7% to 9% to around 2% to 3%. This underscores the urgency in seeking medical help, making a prompt diagnosis, and immediate mechanical intervention in the cardiac catheterization laboratory to unclog the artery. This must be done within 90 minutes to preserve heart muscle and protect lives. That involves increased public awareness of the urgency and heart attack symptoms, an emergency medical team (EMT) that understands the problem, and transporting a suspected heart attack patient to an appropriate facility that has a round-the-clock rapid response team to get the patient into the cardiac catheterization laboratory and unclog the artery.

Public education: Not all chest pains mean a heart attack, but the ones that result from a heart attack need immediate attention. How can we tell the difference? Sometimes it is impossible to tell the difference without appropriate tests, which can only be done in a hospital setting. Any sudden chest pain or discomfort that lasts more than ten minutes should be of concern and needs immediate attention. If you have associated sweating, dizziness, or weakness, you need help. Sometimes the pain could be just below the rib cage, which can be confusing. If you have similar symptoms, or if you are not sure, the best advice is to get someone else to rush you to the nearest emergency center, preferably to one that is equipped to handle heart attack patients in an expeditious manner. These symptoms in a patient with previous heart disease should also signal urgency in seeking medical help. If you cannot get someone to take you to a hospital, call 911.

Emergency medical team: As we understand and underscore the urgency in treating a heart attack patient, we need a knowledgeable and qualified EMT responding to 911 calls from chest pain patients. The EMT should be able to reach the site in a swift manner and diagnose the problem. Present-day technology can enable an EMT to get a 12-lead electrocardiogram on-site and send it to a hospital facility that has the rapid response team to handle such emergencies. The EMT also needs education in recognizing EKG abnormalities related to a heart attack and anticipate the immediate complications such as arrhythmias or drop in blood pressure. They need to have the resources to treat the patients until they arrive at a hospital facility. Also, the EMT needs to be familiar with facilities that have rapid response teams, including the routes they have to take during peak and off-peak hours to transport heart attack patients in a timely manner. This requires city management, the EMT, and nearby hospitals to work in concert.

Hospital rapid response team: It takes tremendous resources to create, establish, and manage a rapid response team to deal with heart attack patients year-round. It involves informed emergency personnel, qualified cardiologists and cardiac surgeons, a ready cardiac surgery team, and a round-the-clock operational cardiac catheterization laboratory with trained people. It needs an administrative team that is willing to commit time, personnel, and finances to see the system performs with laser precision at all levels.

It involves a more coordinated team effort than a symphony orchestra. In a symphony, everything is choreographed, rehearsed, and etched on music sheets. And, above all, you have a conductor to keep things in order and motion. Here, we have teams with different members who do things differently on broad general scheme of action plans. The problems are unknown at the offset, and the treatment options are highly variable, from doing nothing to performing a coronary intervention with a stent or sending a patient for emergency heart surgery in the face of a major heart attack. All patients get an EKG in the emergency room, aspirin, and in most cases, a blood thinner such as Plavix. You may also receive morphine for pain and oxygen before you are transported to the cardiac catheterization laboratory.

Finally, as an educated healthcare consumer, you need to know that time is heart muscle and life. You need to know when to seek help, where to go, and where you have the best survival chance. The next time you visit your family doctor or your cardiologist, be sure to ask these prudent questions.

Sudden Cardiac Death

Sudden cardiac death is a major health problem which most people think may not concern them. Each year, more than 300,000 people die suddenly following a major heart attack, even before they get medical help. The real challenge to patients and medical professionals is to identify who is at risk for sudden death and what can be done to prevent such an unfortunate incidence. We have come a long way in identifying what causes sudden death, who is at a higher risk for such events, and what treatment options are available to prevent such events.

What is sudden cardiac death? A person who has a heart attack can develop a fatal cardiac rhythm disturbance known as ventricular fibrillation or chaotic rhythm, where the heart is not able to pump any blood. If this is not promptly treated with defibrillation and medications, the person can develop cardiac arrest, which can lead to sudden death. Rarely, some people may develop severe slowing of the heart rate to the point where life is not sustainable.

The main function of the heart is to pump blood to the rest of the body and to maintain brain function. When there is major damage to the heart muscle, the heart loses its pumping efficiency and fails to deliver the required amount of blood to the brain and other organs. When the blood supply to the brain is cut off for four minutes or longer, the brain suffers permanent damage.

What are the other causes of sudden death? People can die suddenly from causes other than a heart attack. Some people may have a weakness in the aortic wall that can lead to a split or tear in the aortic lining, which can cause sudden death. Massive stroke can also lead to sudden death. People who have a tendency for blood clot formation may develop massive clots that can lodge in the lung blood vessels and cause pulmonary embolism, which can rarely cause sudden death. Sometimes, we hear of athletes dying suddenly on the field, which may be related to hypertrophy, or thickening of the heart muscle. An intense adrenaline surge also has been shown to be associated with sudden cardiac death. Certain drugs such as cocaine and others can cause a severe coronary artery spasm that can lead to heart attack and sudden death.

Who is at risk for sudden cardiac death? There are certain conditions that can greatly increase the risk of sudden death. People who have a history of previous heart attack and a heart pumping function of less than 30% (normal pumping function is between 55% to 70%) are at increased risk of developing serious arrhythmias that can lead to sudden death. Therefore, people with congestive heart failure or cardiomyopathy (enlarged and flabby heart with weak function) are at increased risk. People who also exhibit significant rhythm disturbances such as ventricular tachycardia or fibrillation are also at increased risk of sudden cardiac death. Ironically, sudden death may be the first symptom of heart disease in some people. Interestingly, 90% of the people who die suddenly have been found to have two- or three-vessel coronary artery disease. That underscores the important relationship between coronary artery disease and sudden cardiac death.

Can we revive a person who has undergone cardiac arrest? The most common finding during a cardiac arrest is a serious rhythm disorder such as ventricular tachycardia or fibrillation that ceases the blood circulation. So the immediate concern during a cardiac arrest is to establish circulation by restoring a normal heart rhythm. If a person is having a ventricular fibrillation, the first step is to initiate cardiopulmonary resuscitation (CPR) by pumping on the chest at a rate of 60 to 80 beats per minute, while someone gets a defibrillator ready, if one is available. As soon as the defibrillator is available, the heart must be defibrillated to restore normal rhythm. If a defibrillator is not available, continue manual CPR until medical help arrives.

What are the ABCs of basic cardiac life support? If you are in a situation where someone collapses, what do you do? Do not panic.

First, yell "Help, someone has fallen unconscious."

Next, shake the person and ask, "Are you OK?"

People may pass out for various reasons. If the person had a common faint, soon after hitting the floor, that person may be beginning to regain consciousness. If you are familiar with the ABCs of basic life support, you might have a chance to save the life of a person who has had a cardiac arrest.

The letter "A" stands for "airway." You extend the person's neck to open up the airway and make sure the tongue is not blocking the airway.

The letter "B" stands for "breathing." If the person is not breathing, you deliver two quick breaths using mouth-to-mouth resuscitation or a mouthpiece.

The letter "C" stands for "circulation." Now, you try to establish the presence of adequate circulation. You do this by placing the fingertips on the neck, over the carotid artery, to feel for the carotid pulse. If you feel a pulse, determine whether the pulse is strong or weak. If the pulse is very weak or if there is no pulse, the amount of blood pumped by the heart maybe inadequate. If you feel the circulation is not adequate and the person appears dusky or blue because of lack of oxygen, begin cardiac compressions.

You place the base of your palm over the lower part of the chest, just above the belly, and reinforce it with the other hand. You compress the chest about an inch with your upper body weight delivering the pressure and force. Continue these chest compressions at a rate of 60 to 80 per minute. After every 15 to 20 compressions, perform a quick pulse check, deliver two breaths and continue with the chest compressions.

What is beyond the basic CPR? We need to go beyond the

basic life support measures in a true cardiac arrest to fully resuscitate a person. The most important thing to address is what caused the cardiac arrest to begin with, namely ventricular fibrillation. That can be treated with automatic defibrillators. That is one reason that airlines and schools are required to have defibrillators that can be used in times of emergency. Certain drugs are essential in treating slow heart rhythms and preventing recurrent ventricular fibrillation.

How do we identify and treat people with increased risk of sudden cardiac death? The first step is to identify people with risk factors for heart disease, such as high cholesterol, diabetes, hypertension, smoking, and family history of heart disease. They need to undergo thorough cardiac evaluation including echocardiogram, nuclear stress test, and even coronary angiograms if indicated. They need appropriate treatment and follow-up to reduce their risk factors and watch for early signs of heart disease. The treatment options available include medicines for irregular heart rhythms and high cholesterol. Coronary angioplasty or bypass surgery for critical blockages may be needed.

People with heart attacks and poor heart function need special attention. Preventive (prophylactic) placement of an implantable defibrillator (a pacemaker that can defibrillate the heart if there is an irregular rhythm--an ICD) has been shown to reduce the incidence of sudden cardiac death in this high risk group.

Sudden cardiac deaths can happen to people with no history of heart disease. Therefore, the knowledge of basic life support may help you save someone's life. Prompt CPR can double or triple the rate of survival in cardiac arrest victims.

Chapter 20

Anxiety, Stress & Depression

Anxiety & Panic Attacks

Did you ever walk into a room and suddenly feel bewildered, with your heart racing, hands shaking, and body perspiring? Were you feeling dizzy or fuzzy, with a sinking sensation? Did you ever notice weakness in your legs? And a smothering sensation, or that you were about to pass out? If so, you are not alone. There are millions of people who go through similar experiences from time to time at a school, church, shopping mall, or in other crowded places, even in the sanctity of their own home. For some, these symptoms may be so severe that they may not be able to carry on their daily activities. The above described symptoms are an example of a panic attack.

Then, there are others who have a general anxiety or nervousness for years, and get hooked on prescription pills, alcohol, drugs, or cigarettes to suppress their symptoms. They also experience nervousness, palpitation, sweating, and some dizziness, but not to the extent experienced by people with panic attacks. Chronic anxiety may indeed be an external expression of a mild depression.

Panic attacks and anxiety disorders may be related to a family history, a past traumatic experience, a bad relationship, stress at the workplace, a financial crisis, or other situations. It may also represent an emotional problem, where an individual dreads facing a situation and gets obsessed and overwhelmed by all the things that can go wrong. That person may exhaust all energy in these negative thoughts, thus allowing no time for the mind to respond normally to a simple challenge. As a result, the person may feel very nervous, weak, and dizzy, and may experience all other panic symptoms just thinking of the dreaded outcome, which often never happens.

Most people with panic disorder or anxiety go through life re-creating the unpleasant past and dreading the future. They never have time to live in the present.

Some panic or anxiety symptoms may be simply related to a normal fight response, where your body releases adrenaline, which increases the heart rate and respiration and causes flushing. On the other hand, a flight (fear) response is associated with slow heart rate, weakness in the legs, and a sensation of being about to faint. These symptoms are an expression of slowing of the heart rate and pooling of the blood in the lower extremities. There may be strong emotional components that can repeatedly trigger these hormonal responses to even simple situations.

Some people with depression may have low levels of a brain neurotransmitter called serotonin, which acts as a link between nerve cells and helps them to transmit information and communicate with one another. Replacing serotonin has been found useful in controlling depression and anxiety symptoms.

Treatment of Panic Attacks

The key is to understand what is precipitating your attacks. You need to make a note of those situations that provoke your attacks and how your mind and body respond to those situations. Keep a notebook and list all the symptoms that you feel before, during, and after an anticipated attack. Usually, the symptoms begin long before you face a stressful situation. Keep a note of a stressful situation that may bring on your panic or anxiety attacks. List all the abnormal things you feel: heart rate, respiration, sweating, dizziness, fuzziness, spaced-out feeling, hot sensation, or anything else. You may feel these symptoms several times before the dreaded incidence, but don't worry. The symptoms may even intensify as you get closer to the situation. Once you confront the dreadful situation, your anxiety level may indeed be a little less. Engage your mind in the act of dealing with the situation and the solution to the problem. That leaves very little room for negative thoughts. When the situation has come to pass and none of the dreaded outcomes has happened, you are relieved. You feel like you could have walked through the situation after all, without any sweat. The key to successful treatment of panic and anxiety attacks is to feel good, enthusiastic, and optimistic before you face a given situation so that you can put your best effort at facing it. Focus all your energy on dealing with the situation, and come out feeling better, satisfied, and exhilarated, not feeling drained or exhausted.

Panic attacks and anxiety are multi-factorial, meaning they may be related to hormonal, physical, emotional, or personal causes, or to chemical imbalances in the brain. Therefore, a multi-pronged approach is essential in dealing with these situations. It may take a long time to gain confidence and overcome fear and anxiety.

Since most physical manifestations of panic attacks are related to adrenaline or hormones related to vagal nerve stimulation, they can be controlled by reprogramming our minds, our perception of the challenges, and our response to a given stress, which leads to the decreased release of these agents in the body.

Exercise also helps to reduce our body's response by releasing lesser amounts of adrenaline for a given level of stress. We also need to minimize our focus on these hormonal surges. As time goes on, your body will learn not to respond to every simple thought with a burst of adrenaline. It is like developing immunity to minimally negative thoughts that never really harm anyone in the long run.

Meditation is an excellent way to suppress your body's response to hormonal surges and engage your mind positively. As I mentioned, the moment your mind perceives an idea of facing a dreaded situation, it will shift the negative thoughts into overdrive. If you force your mind to focus on meditation and chant the word "Om," or something else that soothes your mind, now literally you have put your negative thoughts on hold. That will reduce your body's adrenaline surges. As you focus on the meditation, slow your breathing. Taking deep breaths in and out will help to reduce your hyperventilation. When your breathing turns normal, your dizziness becomes less obvious. These may sound too good to be true. And, you are right! It takes much practice, and therefore, maintaining a diary is important to chart your course.

Knowledge is power. It provides confidence and insight. So, reading a couple of books on these topics might shed some light on how experts have approached these problems in a systematic manner that can greatly benefit you.

Imagery is a useful way to redirect your mind away from negative thoughts. I use this technique whenever I am doing stress tests or heart catheterizations on patients. I tell my patients to imagine that they are lying on a beach in Hawaii, watching a beautiful sunset, while sipping their favorite drink and enjoying the fireworks. You can create your own imagery or recall a pleasant or a funny incident in your life, and slowly, replay the act, one step at a time, enjoying every moment. By all means, take your time.

You also need to get plenty of sleep. If you cannot sleep because your mind is in overdrive with negative thoughts, try reading a book, drinking warm milk (no caffeine), or taking a hot shower.

People with mixed anxiety and depression may have a chemical imbalance in the brain that may respond to serotonin releasing drugs. There are natural substances that can work on people with mild depression. One such agent is St. John's wort. The active ingredient in this plant increases serotonin levels in the brain and helps to control the symptoms of mild depression and anxiety. Similarly, 5-hydroxytrytophan (5-HTP) also increases brain serotonin levels and improves symptoms in mild depression cases.

In resistant and persistent cases, a more challenging part is addressing the emotional aspect, which requires the help of a trained professional who is well versed in cognitive behavioral therapy.

Stress Response

Let us imagine for a moment that you are in line for that long-awaited job interview. You desperately need that job, and you are nervous about the interview. You are trying to put on your best front, while your heart is racing, respiration is labored, and sweat is ruining your clothes. You have already made your third trip to the restroom and are wondering why the room feels hot. Do not despair. This is just your body's "fight response" to an anticipated stressful situation.

Now consider another individual who is called upon to speak in front of 300 people. This person, who is facing the greatest fear known to the human race, namely, public speaking, suddenly notices weakness in the legs, dizziness, mental confusion, and shakiness. That person may be thinking, "I'd rather be dead than making a speech in front of 300 people." This is the "flight response" to a very stressful circumstance.

What is stress? It is the body's reaction to internal or external environmental changes or challenges. These reactions are due to the autonomic nervous system, which either increases adrenaline production or releases a hormone called acetylcholine through the vagal nerve. People who respond by an adrenaline surge display the fight symptoms such as palpitation, sweating, and rapid respiration. Acetylcholine released during the vagal stimulation produces the flight symptoms such as slowing of the heart rate, even stopping of it for several seconds, a drop in blood pressure, and dizziness or fainting. The underlying sequence of events leading to this is very complex and involves our psychological, mental, emotional, and physical make-up, prior exposure, and experience with similar situations.

Stress management: Make a list of situations that are stressful to you, how your body responds to those situations, and what makes you nervous. Be aware that 99% of the wrong things that we imagine never happen in real life. Therefore, direct most of your effort and energy on positive thoughts, while keeping in mind the chances of a bad outcome are very slim, and you are prepared to deal with the unexpected by anticipation and continuing training. When you face an unpleasant situation, it is not the time to wonder why it is happening to you, who is responsible for this, etc. This is the perfect time to face the situation, do your best, and worry later about what you need to do to improve your performance in the future.

The body's response to stress is multi-factorial and therefore, we need a multidisciplinary approach to address its physical, mental, emotional, psychological, and personal effects. The following is a partial list of things that you may consider as you prepare to face your stress.

Communication: This is the link that binds us with the people around us. Learn to effectively get your thoughts across to other people. At the same time, try to understand the other person's views. Highlight the facts while minimizing your emotions.

The art of dynamic listening: It is where you actively engage in understanding the other person's point of view while paying full attention, noting relevant data, asking questions, clarifying issues, and restating what you understand in a summary.

Your attitude: Your attitude in life influences very strongly how you look at the universe and how people around you judge you. You can say, "the glass is half empty," or "the glass is half full." Why not start with the attitude the glass is already half full, and every attempt you make to add a little more will get you ever closer to filling the glass with your rich and colorful life experiences.

Assertive behavior: It is where you make your point in a firm and positive manner without raising your voice or temper. Once you make your point, you should stand by your words and actions.

Time management: Time management can eliminate much stress. It is not the lack of time but the lack of time management that robs our patience. Write down everything you want to carry out in a day including your free time and then add 10% extra time for delays or unexpected tie-ups. If all your activities cannot fit within 24 hours, you need to delete some items on the list or postpone them to another day.

A crisis survival kit: It is like an insurance policy for major stresses in life such as the loss of a loved one, breakups of relationships, or loss of a job, among others. Make a list of things you need to do and how you would address the crisis, and mentally rehearse.

Healthy eating habits: They create a sense of well-being, increase your self-image, and boost your confidence. Everyone knows what good eating habits are, but has trouble starting or staying with them. Let us start with one simple change today and add a few more as time progresses.

Exercise: It is the key to excellence. Exercise conditions your body's response to stress (reduces heart racing), improves your strength and endurance, creates a sense of accomplishment, helps to reduce your weight, brings down blood pressure and lowers cholesterol.

Meditation: It is the ability to control your mind during a stressful situation and direct your mind to focus on solutions rather than problems. Begin by closing your eyes and focusing on an abstract object for a few seconds and then gradually increase the duration.

Imagery: It is an approach that Olympic athletes use as part of their rehearsals in preparation for the finals. You create imagery of a stressful situation from start to finish and experience all the unpleasant things that you might encounter and how you are going to deal with them in a positive problem-solving manner. When you practice this a hundred times, you will be ready to perform what you have already rehearsed.

Relaxation and yoga: They reduce symptoms such as muscle tension associated with stress. Relaxation involves mentally relaxing a group of muscles at will from top to bottom.

Biofeedback: This approach trains your mind to progressively reduce the body's response to stress. This is accomplished by using machines that monitor your heart rate, respiration, sweating, and temperature under imagined stressful situations. Using music, relaxation, and imagery, your mind is trained to influence those responses positively.

A good night's sleep: This is essential before starting a stressful day. Avoid caffeine in the evening. Evening exercise will also help you to get a good night sleep.

Music with 60 beats per minute has been shown to reduce the heart rate, slow respiration, and calm nerves.

Depression & Heart Disease

A lady patient of mine had a heart attack. I thought she was a bit depressed. I sent her to a psychiatrist for evaluation. While the psychiatrist was talking to her, he said, "Ma'am, you've got to quit smoking!"

"Why?" my patient asked with dejection.

"Didn't your heart doctor tell you that smoking is bad for your heart?" he replied.

"I can understand my heart doctor being worried about my smoking. Why are you worried about my smoking?" she asked in an irritated voice.

"Because you're burning my couch!" he replied.

The relationship between smoking and heart disease is much easier to understand and address. However, the relationship between heart disease and depression and vice versa is less recognized and understood, which may have a bearing on how people who have heart disease or depression respond with their depressive or cardiac symptoms. Unfortunately, more than 50% of depressive symptoms go unrecognized.

Depression 101: Depression is a mood disorder where people feel down, sad, and gloomy. Roughly 6% of men and 18% of women in the general population suffer from depression. The prevalence of depression in medically ill patients may be as high as 40%. Family history, physical health, mental state, stress in life, and chemical imbalances in the body can contribute to symptoms of depression. It is not a personal failure or weakness.

The most common symptoms of depression are feeling down or lacking interest in all activities. Other symptoms include a change in appetite, weight, lack of sleep or excess sleepiness, and fatigue or loss of energy. Others include agitation or slowing down, feelings of guilt or worthlessness, inability to think or concentrate, thoughts of death or suicide, unusual tearfulness, social withdrawal, and feeling hopeless or helpless.

Depressive symptoms: Depression can increase the risk of death after a cardiac event. Following cardiac surgery, it can intensify pain, fatigue, hamper recovery because of sluggishness, and promote isolation from society. People may also express hostility and irritability. It also can promote bad habits such as drinking, smoking, and overeating, among others, as a means of coping with the depressive symptoms.

However, when the depressive symptoms last for more than 3 or 4 weeks, and they occur daily, they not only can interfere with recovery, but also can make your symptoms worse. Depression also can increase the chances of blood clots.

Heart disease and depression: Diagnosis of a heart disease, heart attack, or need for heart surgery can send chilling and repelling reactions through that person's mind and have a long-term effect on that person's life. These effects can have an intense influence on that person's ability to return to full functionality.

One out of six people with a heart attack suffer from depressive symptoms. It is not unusual to have some sadness and depressive symptoms after a life changing event such as a heart attack or heart surgery. Generally, these symptoms last only a few weeks.

Depression and heart disease: Patients with a history of depression have an increased risk of developing cardiovascular diseases and increased risk of dying from them. Depression is associated with a worse outcome following a heart attack. Depression is an independent risk factor for future cardiovascular events.

Patients with depression have increased levels of a stress hormone called cortisol, increased platelet stickiness, heart irritability, and elevated blood pressure.

Diagnosis of depression: Every practicing physician should be aware that people are prone to depression after a major illness. A simple questionnaire should bring out certain subtle symptoms that patients may normally not mention. Watch for symptoms such as lack of sleep, inability to concentrate, short temper, irritability, sadness, etc.

Recognizing the presence of depression symptoms is very important from the physician's point of view, which can be accomplished by observation and this simple questionnaire completed by the patient. If there are enough symptoms in favor of a depressive mood, treating these patients with mild antidepressive medicines can help to reduce their depressive symptoms.

Certain medicines can cause symptoms similar to depression. Your physician should be able to identify this possible source of your symptoms by looking at a list of medicines you are on.

Actually, there are no tests designed to diagnose depression. It is recognized by certain symptoms. Therefore, simple screening questions can aid in the diagnosis of depression.

Depression Screening Test

Please answer the following questions:
In the last two weeks, have you experienced any of the following symptoms?

- Depression or loss interest in all activities?
- Change in appetite or weight?
- Insomnia or hypersomia?
- Fatigue or loss of energy?
- Agitation or sluggishness?
- Guilt or worthlessness?
- Inability to think or concentrate?
- Thoughts of death or suicide?
- Unusual tearfulness?
- Social withdrawal?
- Hopelessness or helplessness?

Five symptoms may suggest major depression, while two or three symptoms may signal a minor depression.

Two most important questions that can identify more than 95% of the patients with depression are:

In the past one month, have you felt down, depressed, or hopeless?

In the past one month, have you had little pleasure or interest in doing things?

Depression management: Management of depression is a team effort between the physician and you. Your physician might recommend a combination of psychotherapy (talk sessions) and/or certain antidepressant drugs.

The antidepressant medicines belong to a class of drugs called selective serotonin re-uptake inhibitors (SSRIs), which have been found to be useful in reducing depressive symptoms and are safe to use in cardiac patients. The commonly used drugs in this class include Prozac, Paxil, Zoloft, and Celexa. Wellbutrin (Zyban) and Effexor are useful as a second line of drugs in the treatment of depression in cardiac patients.

Your role in depression treatment: Simple pills are not going to alleviate your depressive symptoms. You have to take a very proactive step toward shifting your lifestyle focus in a positive direction with proper diet, exercise, smoking cessation, weight control, and relaxation, which should provide a more upbeat and optimistic outlook toward your future.

In addition, you might also consider some other measures:

- Get dressed every day
- Take a daily walk
- Join a network of people with similar interests
- Have hobbies
- Increase your social interactions
- Share your feelings with family
- Get a good night's sleep
- Increase your awareness of heart disease and depression
- Take charge in making decisions again

Depressive symptoms may begin showing improvement within 2 to 3 weeks. Research has shown that treating depression does not necessarily reduce cardiovascular events, but it certainly helps you handle the situation in a more positive manner.

In summary, anxiety is a common symptom among heart patients, which can easily be managed with training and understanding. I have discussed several steps on handling your day-to-day anxiety and stress. It is important to recognize symptoms of depression, and get early treatment to improve your well-being.

Chapter 21

Music, Meditation & Sleep

Music

The first note of a song can inspire a nation of people. A sequence of musical notes can bring back decades of memories, and put tears in people's eyes. Music can bring people of all races, ages, and ethnic backgrounds to have an individualized and unique experience. Music is magic, mystic, and has incredible influence on our emotions and physical well-being. Yet, not all music is healthy. Let us take a journey on understanding the effects of various kinds of music on our physical, emotional, and mental aspects of life.

Music, besides being melodious and pleasing to hear, has many health benefits. Music creates vibrations in our mind and body that are similar to its tempo. It has been an integral part of several forms of therapy such as relaxation, accelerated learning, exercise, and entertainment.

Music and discipline: Music also teaches us discipline. It helps us to cultivate a sense of rhythm, timing, sequence, pattern recognition, repetition, precision, and concentration. Children enrolled in music classes can solve math problems involving space and time much easier, as they use the same principles in learning music.

Music and accelerated learning: Music also accelerates learning of foreign languages. Dr. George Lozano, a Bulgarian physician, introduced the theory of accelerated learning using music. Play soothing, slow, and relaxing music while your children do their homework in the house.

Music and stress reduction: Music can bring our heart rate down to as slow as 60 beats per minute or increase our heart rate to 160 beats per minute, in seconds. Music has a powerful effect on our emotions. This principle is useful in treating stress. Largo music, which has a tempo at sixty beats per minute, helps us to relax and bring our heart rate down. This is especially true in those people who experience rapid heartbeats or palpitations during periods of anxiety or stress. Meditation, combined with slow, relaxing largo music, helps us to bring down our blood pressure, decrease respiration, and minimize sweating. Largo music increases the alpha activity of the brain, which is a reflection of a relaxed state of mind. Interestingly, these changes may last long after the music stops.

In essence, it reduces the effects of an adrenaline rush. It also reduces the cortisol (a stress hormone) levels. Therefore, meditation practiced regularly can be very helpful. Listening to slow, relaxing music on the way to a stressful job or an interview might help. You could also play this music in the background at your home or in your office. We have several hours of such recordings, which we play in our office throughout the day.

Classical music with slower tempos is used in operating rooms to reduce stress and help concentration.

Music and exercise: As I mentioned before, our body tries to vibrate at the frequency or the tempo of music being played. So, if you want to exercise, you would like to have music with tempos greater than 100 beats per minute. If you move your body with each beat or pulse, in rhythmic faction, you could not only enjoy the music, but also get your exercise at the same time. Maybe this is a good time to get all your family members involved in this experiment, so they all benefit from the exercise. That is better than all the family members watching a soap opera with a big bag of chips and 32-ounce soft drinks. This also will help you to avoid deadly cigarette smoke and sound pollution that you may have to put up with in the clubs.

Energizing music increases the adrenaline rush and cortisol levels, which inspires players and spectators before the start of a game. Therefore, you may have noticed that a heavy brass band usually plays before opening a high school or professional football game.

Music and public education: Music also can be a very powerful educational tool in inspiring the younger generation. Michael Jackson, the king of pop, who recently passed away at the tender age of 50 years, showed how music could influence generations of people. As I was doing research on this topic, I was very impressed with the influence of hip-hop music all around the world. While we were planning on performing a bhangra hip-hop fusion for our annual gala, we learned that hip-hop was not just an American phenomenon. There is Japanese hip-hop, Chinese hip-hop, French hip-hop, and British hip-hop. Yes, indeed, there is Panjabi hip-hop, Gujarati hip-hop, and a hip-hop song in just about every language you can think off. I want to underscore the importance of hip-hop as a communication language, which can educate teenagers on the dangers of sex, smoking, drugs, and overindulgence in unhealthy foods.

Other benefits: Music therapy has been used in treating cancer patients, children with attention deficit disorder (ADD), depression, as well as for pain. Music also boosts immunity and relax muscles. Music during an active labor and delivery makes the experience a more pleasant one.

Harmful effects of music: Music also has its toll on people. In particular, drummers exposed to loud sounds for years can develop constant ringing in their ears, which may be difficult to get rid of. Listening to loud music through earphones may damage your hearing apparatus and cause hearing loss. Similarly, listening to very loud music in night clubs can damage your ears. Night club music may also inspire you to overindulge in alcohol, and perhaps experiment with drugs.

Make your own music: If you own a classical music collection, you could collect music segments with a largo tempo (60 beats per minute), and record them on a separate CD or an MP3 player so you can listen to them whenever you want. You may have to scan through many CDs to find largo type music, as those segments may last only a few minutes in each recording. You also can record those segments from the Internet, if you can get one of the free audio-recording software packages, which you can find on the Internet. You could also scan music stores for a collection of slow tempo music, which may be labeled as music for relaxation or meditation.

Music and friendship: Make music a hobby. It will help you to interact with like-minded people and expand your horizons. It will help you to meet new people and make new friends in the comfort of your passion. Besides, you will have an enjoyable evening out. Getting out of your closet, going out to a musical function, enjoying the music and friendship, and creating a positive and meaningful experience, are emotionally and physically beneficial.

Music therapy: Music therapy is a science, which involves not only listening to music, but also taking part in creating music, writing lyrics, composing and performing.

Visit the http://www.musictherapy.org/ site to learn more about the benefits of music in your daily life.

Meditation

Imagine traveling back in time to 2000 B.C. You are at the foothills of Mount Everest. You have enjoyed a cold bath in a nearby creek, at the dawn of another beautiful day filled with radiant sunlight. The cool breeze is gently drifting the fragrance of blossoms everywhere. You approach a giant oak tree as you drape your chest with a freshly washed wet saffron cloth. As you settle down on top of your tigerskin mattress, you rest your left arm over a Y-shaped wooden stick. As your long, curled, and knotted hair drapes over your back and beyond, you notice your right-hand finger gently rolling the rose beads one by one. As you point your chin toward the sky, and gaze at the sun with your eyes closed, you begin your mantras. You quickly gravitate into your meditation for the next two decades. You notice a decline in your heart rate, respiration, a dip your body temperature, and a tranquil state of mind, filled with peace and calmness.

What is meditation? It is an ancient art of focusing your attention on a single object so you control your thoughts, mind, and body, including internal organ functions. In other words, with meditation, you can positively change the direction of your mind and body responses to stress. You will develop the ability to slow your heart rate, reduce respiration, minimize sweating, and control your mind and reactions. This newfound power can alter your fight or flight response to stress by replacing it with appropriate actions for a given situation.

An interesting study: While I was making a presentation on meditation, I told my audience, "Let's play a game. I would like you to make a mental note of everything that runs through your mind for the next ten seconds. I will tell you when to start and when to finish." After the study was completed, I asked the audience to recall the thoughts that ran through their minds. One said that a dozen ideas ran through his mind in those ten seconds. I said, "That's good. Most people's minds flash 30 ideas per second during stress. Really, I was testing to see if you could focus your attention on a single object for ten seconds. I know, I did not direct you properly that time. So let's repeat the test again. I want you to focus on a single object for the next ten seconds. Make sure that your mind does not drift away from the object.

At the end of the test time, most people looked frustrated. I asked, "What's the matter?"

They said, "it's hard to do."

"I know," I said, "that is how our mind and brain are programmed from our childhood. We were never taught to concentrate on any single object for an extended period of time."

When I tried this game on my three teenagers, my younger daughter said, "How can your son focus? He has no mind."

I said, "I know. Some people's minds are like a desert—no roses or green leaves, while other people's minds are like jungles, filled with everything."

I encourage you to engage yourself for the next ten seconds in a similar experience. If you, like the rest of us, have trouble focusing your attention on a single object for ten seconds, then you will be fascinated in learning more about the value of meditation.

Dr. Herbert Benson's research: Dr. Benson, a cardiologist from Harvard Medical School, tested the effect of meditation on cardiac patients recovering from heart attacks. He noticed in his patients that meditation was able to bring down their heart rates, lower their respiration, and reduce their blood pressure. As a result, there was a decrease in the body's oxygen consumption and lactic acid production. Brain wave studies showed alpha activity (a sign of relaxation).

Why learn meditation? Unpleasant memories leave indelible scars that repeatedly erupt during stressful periods and engrave new scars. You can bring an end to this cyclic erosion of your sanity with meditation. This allows you to control your mind and thoughts, and redirect them if necessary. It's like erasing everything on your mind and starting with a clean slate.

During periods of crises, your mind tends to wander around like a lost child screaming in search of his mother. Your thoughts, besides sending cold chills through your spine, rob your mind of important time during which you could be intensely focusing on solving one problem after the other.

When you enter a stressful period, your mind engages in a dialogue with your inner voice. Meditation can enable you to shut off your inner voice, the voice that is driven more by the past inadequacies stored in the subconscious mind than by reasoning based on prevailing circumstances. One who fails to reap the benefits of meditation may be condemned to repeat the miserable past.

When you start your meditation practice, you will notice your thoughts slipping out of your mind, like a flower petal gently dropping from your sleepy hands. Our mind flips relentlessly like a tired thin paper strip tied to an electric fan.

A meditation session: Meditation is the practice of focusing your attention on one thing at a time. Often, the meditators repeat a syllable or a word called a mantra. Some people concentrate on their breathing. Whatever object you choose is fine, as long as you can concentrate on that object. Each time your mind drifts from the main focus, remind yourself to concentrate on the original object. When you focus your mind intensely on one object, your mind can't wander into things such as worry, fear, hate, or taxes. Erma Bombeck says that the only time she drifted into any kind of meditation (for a few seconds) was when she paid $30.00 for a Halstone scarf.

To get the maximum benefit from meditation, choose a relatively quiet place, a mental device that provides a constant focus, a comfortable position, and a passive attitude. You can learn to meditate quickly. Initially, you will notice many distractions going through your mind. This is natural and is to be expected. A passive attitude includes a lack of concern about both extrinsic and intrinsic distractions. Initially, learn to meditate for five minutes per day. Then gradually increase the duration of your meditation to 15 or 20 minutes per day. The longer you meditate, the better are the results. While you are meditating, avoid distractions. The benefits of meditation increase with practice. Your attention becomes steadier.

Practice of meditation: First, select a relatively quiet environment, away from the refrigerator or kitchen aromas. Think of a mental device such as a mantra upon which you can intensely focus for a given time. Assume a comfortable body position so that your joints don't freeze before you start the mantra or meditation. Let your body assume a passive attitude by relaxing your muscles. Rid your mind of the delinquent notices from your friendly creditors, and harness the power of your soul over that mantra or object. In doing so, you become one with your mantra.

The second method of meditation involves concentrating on your breathing. Assume a relaxed attitude, close your eyes, and take a few deep breaths. As you inhale and exhale, listen to the rhythmic music of air as it enters and leaves your body. Concentrate on your breathing so that your universal awareness fades into the clouds. Remember, meditation is an acquired skill, and the more you practice, the better you get at it.

The third method of meditation involves fixing your gaze on a single object for a period of time. Assume a relaxed position in a quiet place. Intensely focus your attention on a single object such as a diamond or an almond. Study the shape, size, structure, and the content of that object. Explore the nature of that object and harvest everything related to that object. Try to ignore all the other objects surrounding it. If your mind drifts into something else, try to remind yourself to focus on the target object.

Benefits of meditation: There are times when you need to keep your mind as clear as mountain water. Meditation enables you to focus intensely on a single object during periods of stress so you can move your thoughts from one problem-solving compartment to another. This prevents your mind from engaging in groundless negative thoughts that not only erode your sanity, but also prevent you from dealing with the situation at hand. Therefore, you can translate the practice of a mantra to intensely focus upon anything.

Meditation helps in the treatment of hypertension, heart disease, strokes, migraine headaches, diabetes and autoimmune diseases such as arthritis. People with anxiety, depression, and hostility also benefit from meditation.

When I was trying to inspire my three teenage children to get involved in meditation, they said, "We know what you are trying to do. You don't want to kill us outright! This is one way for you to shut our minds off for a few minutes each day."

I said, "Your minds are never awake when it comes to paying attention to me."

A Good Night's Sleep

Mr. Johnson, a patient of mine, had heart surgery. While I was making my rounds, I asked, "Mr. Johnson, how did you sleep last night?"

"I didn't sleep all night. I was tossing and turning," he said.

"But, Mr. Johnson, the nurse's notes said that you slept very well. You did not even ask for a sleeping pill."

"Whatever!" he said.

The next day, I asked, "Mr. Johnson, how did you sleep last night?"

"I told you, Dr. Nik, I did not sleep all night. I was miserable. Those sleeping pills don't do me any good," he said.

"But, Mr. Johnson, the nurse's notes said that you slept very well."

The third day, I asked the same question. Mr. Johnson replied, "I do not know, Dr. Nik. I will have to check the nurse's notes!"

What is sleep? Sleep is a state of temporary unconsciousness. The Almighty in his infinite wisdom created sleep to bridge the gap between despair and hope. A normal adult usually falls asleep within 5 to 15 minutes of lying down. There are five stages of sleep:

Stage one represents muscle relaxation, drooping of the eyelids, rolling of the eyes, and a decrease in brain wave voltage.

Stage two is characterized by changes in the brain wave patterns.

Stages three and four represent deep sleep.

Stage five, the final stage, involves further muscle relaxation and bursts of rapid eye movements (REM sleep).

The first four stages, also known as the non-REM or NREM, last from 70 to 100 minutes. Both the REM and NREM cycles repeat four to five times during a night. Most complete sleep cycles last 90 to 100 minutes. It is important to keep in mind that if you try to take a nap on Sunday morning in church and have a loud snore, you may run the risk of waking up others.

What changes occur during sleep? Dreams usually occur during the REM sleep cycle. The dreams may be related to something that your mind was working on, or they may be totally unrelated. It is much easier to awaken someone during the NREM sleep cycle than during the REM sleep cycle. It is uncommon to see people in a drenching sweat following a bad dream. There are gross involuntary body movements, which are normal. Overactivity of a certain (aminergic) hormone may cause sleep disturbance. Therefore, an agent such as diazepam that blocks such a hormone may be useful in restoring sleep in some individuals. Similarly, reduced activity of the same hormone could lead to excess sleep, which can be counteracted by stimulants such as amphetamines. However, these amphetamines are sometimes used for excess stimulation and for avoiding sleep during term finals by young people. Some people taking these medicines may experience heartburn at night due to acid reflux into the esophagus. Rarely, some people may experience a sour taste in the mouth, coughing, choking or respiratory difficulty.

What are the effects of sleep loss? Deprived of sleep, laboratory animals have died within a few days, despite being well fed, watered, and housed. In one study, young medical students deprived of sleep for 3 to 4 days experienced increased mental and physical fatigue, irritability, and difficulty concentrating. Their skilled motor activity performance deteriorated. If your partner complains of not having had good sleep for several days, then watch out for these signs and do not let that person get behind the wheel. Occasionally, lack of sleep can unmask psychotic behavior or an irrational temper. Lately, has your boss been acting strange? Why not suggest a sleep vacation.

What are abnormal sleep conditions? Insomnia refers to an inability in initiating and maintaining sound sleep, which could be related to pain, drugs, anxiety, or worry. Sometimes, it may be the first symptom of depression. Caffeine-containing drinks, amphetamines, and cigarettes are some of the causes of insomnia. A new place or having jet lag can also interfere with sleep. This condition responds to a short course of mild sedatives. However, if the condition persists, you need a complete medical checkup.

Narcolepsy is a condition marked by an excessive and uncontrollable tendency to sleep during the daytime. People may fall asleep anywhere and sometimes while they are behind the wheel. Such people may benefit from adrenergic stimulants prescribed by a specialist. Regular sleep at night and proper scheduling of daytime naps may minimize interference with work.

Sleepwalking is a condition where a person during actual sleep may get up and walk around the house, climb stairs, or even cook food. These episodes may last about 15 minutes before they are terminated by returning to bed or awakening. Locking doors and keeping dangerous objects beyond this person's reach may minimize the damage. Some people may be used to talking during sleep. If you are one of those people, you may want to select the words you say, as your spouse may use it against you for the rest of your life.

Sleep apnea, a condition seen in some people, is associated with sleep interrupted many times because of lack of oxygen. It also can cause heart rhythm problems and is usually treated with a breathing machine. Sleep studies can help in the diagnosis of this condition.

How to get a good night's sleep? First, maintain regular sleeping habits. If you go to sleep at 2 in the morning, then you cannot expect to get satisfactory sleep. You will be sleep deprived. Set a time for your sleep depending on when you have to report to work.

You need an adequate amount of sleep. A baby can sleep for 20 hours. A child needs 10 to 12 hours of sleep, and an adult needs 6 to 7 hours of sleep. On the average, women sleep a little more than men.

Avoid taking afternoon naps. It could cost you your job, which can lead to more sleepless nights.

Avoid caffeine late in the evening, as it interferes with sleep. Caffeine is also found in tea, most soft drinks, and cold medicines.

Make sure that you have a firm mattress, and you sleep on the side of the bed that has been assigned to you by your spouse.

Most people feel sleepy after a long day and then get behind the wheel to rush home. If you are too sleepy, take a brief ten minute nap in your office or in the lobby before you hit the road.

Avoid late, heavy, and fatty meals at nighttime. Do not top them off with coffee and alcohol.

Jet lag occurs when we travel abroad, where the time zones are off by several hours. It takes several days for the body to adjust. You can try to adjust to the new time zone by taking a sedative at nighttime in the new place.

Make sure you have completed all your tasks before you go to bed. If you have some unfinished business on your mind, your mind starts to work on it all night. If you have to solve a problem, write down the possible solutions.

Some people take afternoon naps on the weekends to catch up with the sleep they lost during the busy weekdays.

Good exercise in the evening will help you to get a good night's sleep.

Keep the room temperature steady. The early morning hours may have the lowest temperature and a space heater may be useful to keep the temperature steady.

If you cannot sleep, do not force yourself. Get up and do some reading or get busy with an activity. When you are tired, you will fall asleep.

Use sleeping pills very sparingly and only under a physician's guidance. Address the underlying problem that causes the lack of sleep.

Chapter 22

Laughter, the Best Medicine

Humor is a sudden release of built-up tension or surprise. Most humor is derived from an unpleasant or painful experience separated by time and place. When we are experiencing an unpleasant event in life, we feel helpless and humiliated.

Humor is very therapeutic in that it takes us away from reality and makes us feel good. When we laugh, the body releases endorphins that give a natural high. If you can tell jokes and make other people laugh, you get an exhilarating feeling.

If you can collect one joke per day and tell it to your friends, in a couple of years you will have 500 jokes. The best jokes are those which accent the simplest things in real life, in explicit graphic language, as the comedians on Comedy Central do.

***

A lady patient of mine had a heart attack. She came for a follow-up visit. She was a bit under the weather. I made an immediate diagnosis of depression. I sent her to a psychiatrist (AKA, shrink) for evaluation.

While the shrink was talking to her, he said, "Ma'am, you've got to quit smoking!"

"Why?" she asked.

"Because, you are burning my couch!"

***

The other day, I went to a barber shop. The man at the door said, "Sir, have you come here for a haircut or to apply for a job?"

I looked at him again. He said, "Sir, do you want a wig or a perm?"

I said, "Just trim whatever is left in the back of my bald head."

While he was trimming my hair, Jennifer came by. She said, "I can trim your nails for an extra five bucks."

I said, "Go ahead and do it. How much damage can you do for five bucks?"

While she was trimming my nails, I said, "Jennifer, how about you and me go out for dinner?"

"I can't do that, I'm married," she said.

"Why don't you tell your husband that you are going out with your girlfriend?"

She said, "Why don't you! He is standing right behind you, holding the scissors."

***

I have a housekeeper. I've had her for a long time. Anyway, the other day, she said, "Mr. Nikam, your coffee machine-a broke-a, me start clean it. It's broke-a?" in her broken English.

I said, "What did you say?

She said, "Your coffee machine broke-a, not work-a, anymore."

I said, "Just throw it in the garbage."

She said, "Me take-a your coffee machine-a, me home."

I said, "No! You are not going to take my coffee machine to your home!"

She said, "Come on, Mr. Nikam, coffee machine broke-a, no work-a! Me take-a home."

I said, "Fine, fine, take it. Go, go, go."

She said, "Thank you, Mr. Nikam. Thank you, thank you. Now, me go clean your big TV."

I said, "No! Don't touch my TV!"

***

I went to see patient of mine in the hospital who had heart surgery. As soon as I walked in the room, the patient said, "Hi, Dr. Nik, could you please write me a prescription for some cigarettes? This young nurse says that I cannot smoke. I thought you said you fixed my heart."

"You must be out of your mind, I am not going to write you any prescription for cigarettes," I said.

"In that case, I am going to roll 'em with all your doctor's bills and start smokin' up!'

And the nurse said, "Oh, ho! You'll be smoking for a long time, perhaps until your next surgery!"

***

"According to the latest American statistics, 50% of the marriages in this country end in divorce, while the other 50% fight it 'til the bitter end. That is what I call a challenge in life," Charlie Jarvis, a good friend of mine, said.

In the Desi culture, it is more like a 2 to 5% divorce rate, while the remaining 95% fight it 'til the bitter end and that is what I call a real marriage.

***

This lady goes to the cemetery. She is crying. She tells the caretaker, "I can't find him."

"Find whom?" the caretaker said.

"My husband. We buried him last week. There was a huge crowd, a tent, and flowers. I can't find his plot."

The caretaker said, "Ma'am, I have the entire cross-section of the cemetery right here. Just give me his name, I will walk you right through to his plot."

"Webster, Harry Webster."

"Well, let me see. Webster. Webster. Webster? We don't got a Harry Webster. The only Webster we have is Dorothy Webster."

She said, "That's him. I forgot everything is in my name now."

***

This 17-year-old teenage girl asks, "Dad, can I borrow your Mercedes? I want to go to Galveston with my friends."

The dad said, "Are you crazy? I am not going to give you my Mercedes. Miss, you just got your license two months ago."

The daughter was very polite and nice. She said, "That is all right, Dad, if you do not want to give me your car, that is your decision, I respect your decision."

The dad said, "Thanks for being so understanding."

The teenager said, "No problem, dad, but I just want you to remember that 20 years from now, I am going to decide which nursing home you go to."

Dad said, "Make sure you bring the car back home by 10 pm."
***

The other day, the telephone rang at my house. I picked up the phone and said, "Who is this?"

"What do you mean, who is this? This is your daughter who left for college two weeks ago!"

"Really, you sure sound different this time," I said.

"I know, I need more money this time!"

If you want to hear a 30-minute segment of my jokes on an MP3, send me an email.

Ventriloquist Raj & Nik

Life is like a candle in the desert or in the middle of an ocean. Let us enjoy while the flame is still flickering.

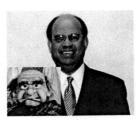

I was thinking, what is the best way to address a group of doctors using humor? One thought that came to my mind was to use a ventriloquist to have a frank, vibrant, and witty dialogue sprinkled with some message, hope, and laughter.

Nik will be conversing with Raj, the ventriloquist's buddy, who is in his mid-60s, with scattered silver hair, a bald head, spectacles, and sharp, uncompromising language.

Nik: Hi, ladies and gentleman, I brought with me today my good old friend Raj. Hi Raj, how do you feel today?

Raj: I don't feel good.

Nik: Why not? You are surrounded by the most educated, intellectual, optimistic and hard-working group of people.

Raj: Because of that, I don't feel good. I feel like I don't belong here. I'm neither intelligent nor hard working. I feel like the engineer who was married to a lady doctor, whose main job is to take care of the kids and do the dishes. Looks like that gentleman knows what I'm talking about (Looking at the audience). Sir, you are laughing your heart out, are you an engineer?

Nik: Come on, you are being cynical. Did you have a good time at the cocktail hour?

Raj: Since my doctor told me that I can't drink, it was like an unhappy hour on a dry, hard rock of ice.

Nik: Really?

Raj: No, on second thought, it was as soft and tasteless as a caffeine-free diet soda.

Nik: So, why are you depressed?

Raj: If you listened to the conversation at that unhappy cocktail hour, you too would be depressed. Talking about cutting someone's gut, while grinding a chicken tikka in the mouth. This lady was on her third samosa, asking her friend whether her competition was looking slimmer than her. I overheard a conversation where one doctor said that he was working all his life for his wife who was living expensively to keep up with her friend, who was living expensively to keep up with her. Oh, I cannot go on.

Nik: You still did not answer my question. Why are you depressed?

Raj: I don't know. Maybe because I'm not a doctor!

Nik: Well, why didn't you go to medical school?

Raj: If only I had gotten a better score on my SAT test.

Nik: What was your score?

Raj: ZERO! Ah, ha! Zero, like a big, fat 'O.'

Nik: How the hell did you get a zero, Raj?

Raj: They did not explain that on the report card. I think I forgot to sign my name. By the way, I recognize that lady in the red sari.

Nik: She is a doctor.

Raj: She looks familiar.

Nik: Where did you see her?

Raj: I don't know.

Nik: Think hard.

Raj: I think she's the one who delivered me. Yes, she's the one who delivered me.

Nik: Come on. That is the most bizarre thing I have ever heard. Was she younger than you when she delivered you?

Raj: If you don't believe me, I have a tattoo on my behind from her three fingers.

Nik: Where did you come up with this weird theory?

Raj: I'm positive. When I was born, she spanked my rear end, cut off my oxygen cord, and said, 'you are on your own from now on, baby.'

Nik: Raj, do you have a family doctor?

Raj: While my family doctor was checking my lungs, he said, 'cough, cough, cough.'

Nik: Then?

Raj: I coughed, coughed, and coughed.

Nik: Ah, ha.

Raj: He asked, 'How long did you have this stupid cough?' (Looking at the audience) You don't happen to have a cigarette, do you, sir... ma'am?

Nik: Cigarette? These are doctors, they don't smoke!

Raj: You're wrong.

Nik: At your age, shouldn't you be more concerned about cancer and heart disease?

Raj: Speaking of my heart, on my first visit to a heart specialist, he said that I have excess weight, diabetes, high blood pressure, heart failure, high cholesterol, and irregular heart rhythm.

Nik: That's not bad; he saved you money on multiple office visits. What else did he tell you?

Raj: He said, 'Not bad for an 85-year-old man.' I told him that I was only 65.

Nik: Really?

Raj: He said if I were a car or an airplane, he would have recommended me for a junk yard.

Nik: Oh, no! What else did he advise you?

Raj: He said, 'No more smoking, drinking, and cursing.'

Nik: That's it?

Raj: Wait, he said, no samosas, chicken curry, rice, or gulab jamun.

Nik: What's left?

Raj: He said salad and jogging. When I look at all these doctors, it reminds me of those painful visits and depressed moments. Every time you see a specialist, he will make up a new diagnosis if you don't have one.

Nik: Would you like to ask these doctors any questions? Maybe you can squeeze in a free consultation, while they are laughing.

Raj: Did any of you, by any chance, bring some Viagra samples?

Nik: Raj, you are a dirty old man.

Raj: Do not interrupt me...

Nik: You are embarrassing me. I still cannot believe that you would announce in front of more than 500 people that you are looking for help. Are you out of your mind?

NIKAM

Raj: You don't understand. When you get to my age, everybody needs help. When you reach the metallic age, like I have, with silver hair, gold teeth, steel coronary stents, and a titanium hip, you too may use all the help you can get!

Nik: Stop, stop! Didn't you say you have heart disease? If you take Viagra with heart medicines such as nitrates, it could kill you.

Raj: I'd rather take that chance than go home and listen to the music and get more depressed.

Nik: I am baffled by your performance today. Wait till your wife hears this.

Raj: Don't worry about her. She is the one who told me that since I was going to a doctors' convention, to make sure that I get some help. If I come home without it, then I will have one more reason for my depression.

Nik: Do you have any advice for these doctors?

Raj: Please don't think of your patients as ATM machines. Can we get five minutes of your undivided attention, please? You're the only hope we've got. Do not make your patients feel more depressed when they leave your office than they were when they came to see you.

Nik: Raj, you keep mentioning the word "depressed" in front of more than 500 doctors. You will be like a perfect target, a sitting duck for them. Next, they are going to strap you to a stretcher and deliver electric shocks.

Raj: Oh, no, I am not going to go through that again! I was just emphasizing how non-medical people feel when they interact with doctors. Why is that man walking toward me? He's holding something in his hand.

Nik: Just relax; he is the president. Perhaps he is coming to congratulate and thank you.

Raj: Or perhaps, he is coming to electrocute me and my depression. I am a jolly good fellow, I am a jolly good fellow. I am the happiest man around here, and I am a jolly good fellow. Happy holidays! Good night, everybody. Let's get out of here.

Nik: Happy holidays! Good night, everybody!

Chapter 23

Cardiac Arrhythmias

Palpitations

Did you ever have a funny feeling in your chest or a flip-flop in your heart? You could be having a palpitation or extra heartbeat.

Extra heartbeats are very common, and they could be benign. If you pay close attention to your heart rhythm, you may notice that from time to time it may appear that your heart is skipping a beat. In reality, it may be having an extra beat followed by a pause that creates the break in the rhythm, giving the sensation of a flip-flop.

Where do the extra heartbeats come from? The extra heartbeats or contractions can arise from anywhere in the heart. When they arise from the atria (the upper chambers of the heart), they are called atrial premature contractions (PACs); when they arise from the ventricles (the lower chambers of the heart), they are labeled ventricular premature contractions (PVCs). Occasionally, when they arise from the atrio-ventricular node (located at the junction of the upper and lower chambers of the heart), they are termed junctional premature contractions (JPCs).

What causes these extra beats or contractions? The extra beats can result from various conditions. Most of the time, they may not have any significant identifiable causes. The most common cause of having PACs or PVCs in a younger population is mitral valve prolapse (MVP). It is a condition where the mitral valve is floppy. Other medical conditions such as thyroid hormone imbalance, congestive heart failure or coronary artery disease are common among older patients.

What makes these better or worse? Many situations can make these extra beats occur more frequently. Aggravating factors such as smoking, alcohol, drugs, stimulants, and caffeine, among others, can make them worse. Any harmless extra beat frequency should generally decrease during exercise. If your extra beats get worse during exercise, it may warrant further cardiac evaluation. Electrolyte imbalances such as low potassium or magnesium also can lead to or aggravate these extra heartbeats. Patients taking water pills should be particularly aware of this situation, as water pills can reduce both the serum potassium and magnesium levels. Therefore, it is very important to routinely monitor blood chemistries to ensure their levels are optimal. Exhaustion and lack of sleep also can make these extra beats worse. Some cold medicines that contain pseudoephedrine can also precipitate these extra heartbeats.

How do we diagnose these extra heartbeats? People who are having these extra heartbeats can easily feel them. Occasionally, some people are so concerned about these extra beats, they can feel each one. Others may describe them as a strong extra thump in the heart area. Some people may especially feel this regular or irregular skipping of the heartbeat when they are sleeping or in a quiet room. Occasionally, these symptoms may get worse when people are anxious or tense. Yet others may describe these as painful episodes. However, there is no correlation between how people feel and the extent and the frequency of extra heartbeats. Rarely, some people may be totally unaware of their extra heartbeats until they are pointed out by their physicians.

The causes of extra heartbeats can be varied, and therefore the diagnosis of palpitations or extra heartbeats can be challenging and at times frustrating. The diagnostic approach also depends on the underlying causes and the patient's age. Younger individuals are more likely to have a harmless (benign) condition compared with the older population, where coronary artery disease and congestive heart failure are very common causes of extra heartbeats.

The diagnosis begins with careful listening to (auscultation of) the heart. Just by listening, we may not be able to diagnose the exact origin of the extra heartbeats. However, that should alert your physician to further evaluate for any underlying heart disease.

A simple electrocardiogram may pick up these extra heartbeats. When these extra heartbeats occur more often than six times per minute they are considered to be significant. The electrocardiogram will enable us to determine the site of origin of these extra heartbeats.

A 24-hour Holter (EKG) monitor will help us not only in identifying these extra heartbeats, but also in determining the frequency of these extra heartbeats. It can actually measure the number of extra heartbeats in any given 24 hour period. This will enable us to determine the presence of, the frequency, and the severity of these extra heartbeats. It also will help us in evaluating the response to treatment in terms of reduction in the frequency of extra heartbeats after the beginning of a treatment.

An echocardiogram may reveal the presence of any structural abnormalities of the heart that could account for the extra heartbeats. The most common cause in the younger population will be the presence of mitral valve prolapse. It will also enable us to determine the presence of congestive heart failure or abnormal scars that may signal coronary artery disease.

A blood test may enable us to determine any abnormalities in the electrolytes such as calcium, potassium, and magnesium. It will also help us to diagnose any changes in the thyroid hormone levels.

In older patients with multiple risk factors for heart disease, a stress test may help us to identify the presence of any coronary artery disease, which may be the cause of extra heartbeats.

Occasionally, we have to perform an electrical study (electrophysiology or EP study) of the heart to determine the exact site of origin of these extra heartbeats.

Using a radiofrequency wave at the tip of a wire, we can place the wire tip at the site of origin of these extra beats and burn a very tiny area, which will prevent the firing of these extra beats. You may have heard the term radiofrequency ablation used for such a procedure.

What is the prognosis of these extra heartbeats? That depends on the underlying condition causing these extra heartbeats. In a younger individual with no significant underlying heart condition, the prognosis is good. On the other hand, for someone with congestive heart failure or coronary artery disease, the prognosis is related to their underlying heart condition.

How do we treat these extra heartbeats? There are three main issues that we need to address: symptoms related to extra heartbeats, the aggravating factors, and any underlying heart disease.

The symptoms can be very disturbing to some patients. If they have no underlying heart disease, they need reassurance, and if the symptoms are a major concern, a mild tranquilizer may help. We also need to understand that these symptoms may come and go.

The treatment of underlying heart disease is essential to minimize these extra heartbeats and symptoms related to them. We need to be aware of the fact these extra heartbeats reduce the overall heart function and controlling them will not only improve the symptoms but also strengthen overall heart performance.

Finally, we need to address any aggravating factors such as smoking, alcohol, and caffeine, among others. If you eliminate these cardiac stimulants and your symptoms of extra heartbeats disappear, you have one more reason to get rid of your bad habits. Supplements such as fish oil or flaxseeds that are rich in omega-3 fatty acids also reduce certain cardiac rhythm problems.

Most importantly, you need regular follow-up with your physician, who can monitor your symptoms and aggravating factors, then adjust your treatment accordingly.

Atrial Fibrillation

Atrial fibrillation (AF) is one of the most common cardiac arrhythmias or irregular heart rhythms; it is seen in 2.2 million people in the United States. It is the most puzzling problem for both the physician and the patient.

This irregular cardiac rhythm arises from the upper chambers of the heart, namely the atria. The atria beat faster than 350 times per minute, while the ventricles beat at 60 to 150 times per minute. The difference between the rates at which the upper and lower heart chambers beat reduces the pumping efficiency of the heart. That is just one of the problems related to this rhythm disturbance.

Causes of AF: The most common cause of AF is coronary artery disease, and it shows up in people over the age of 50 to 60 years. Occasionally, it also can occur in younger individuals without coronary artery disease. Valvular heart diseases such as mitral stenosis, mitral regurgitation, or aortic stenosis stretch the atrial chambers (cavities), which can cause AF. Most patients with congestive heart failure develop AF. It is also seen in almost 30% of the people who undergo heart surgery. Other conditions causing AF include hypertension, thyroid disease, and emphysema.

Symptoms: Some people may experience a sudden onset of AF without any warning. Others may notice palpitations or rapid heartbeats. When they visit their physicians, their EKG may reveal irregular heart rhythm. Occasionally, some may have no symptoms and a routine EKG may unravel the arrhythmia. With reduced heart function, patients may present with worsening heart failure symptoms. In older patients, the AF may be associated with slow ventricular rates, a condition known as the sick sinus syndrome. These patients may notice weakness, lack of energy, dizziness, and fainting episodes. Very rarely, patients may develop blood clots that can cause stroke or lack of circulation in the legs, creating an emergency.

Diagnosis: Routine EKG may reveal AF. It will also establish the ventricular rate, which can be as low as 30 to 40 or as high as 150 to 170 beats per minute. Cardiac enlargement may be noted on examination and chest X-ray. Echocardiogram may confirm the presence of cardiac enlargement, especially of the left atrium, from where most AF arises.

Medical treatment: Most patients can be managed with medicines to control the heart rhythm and sometimes to convert it to a regular rhythm. The chances of conversion to normal sinus rhythm are good if the AF has been in existence for less than a year. The most common drugs used to control the rate include digoxin, beta-blockers such as atenolol and metoprolol, calcium channel blockers such as diltiazem and verapamil, or other drugs such as flecainide and propafenone. These drugs have to be taken on a long-term basis. These drugs also help to maintain sinus rhythm after conversion or interventions. They may at times slow the heart rate to the point where patients may require a pacemaker. When these drugs are ineffective, more expensive medicine such as amiodarone is considered. Amiodarone, though well tolerated, may occasionally cause scarring of the lung tissue (lung fibrosis).

People with AF along with left atrial enlargement have a tendency to develop blood clots in the atria. These blood clots can travel to other regions in the body and block a tiny artery, which can result in loss of circulation. In the brain that can lead to a stroke. Therefore, these patients may be advised to stay on a long-term blood thinner such as warfarin. They need constant monitoring to ensure the blood does not get too thin, potentially leading to serious bleeding. Patients under the age of 75 with low risk factors may be treated with aspirin alone.

Cardioversion: Cardioversion is a technique where an electrical shock is applied to the chest to restore normal heart rhythm. The electrical shock stops all heart rhythms for a couple of seconds and allows the normal rhythm to resume. Patients are usually sedated so that they may not feel or remember the procedure.

People with AF of less than one year without other significant cardiac problems may be candidates for cardioversion to revert the rhythm back to normal. These patients are lightly sedated. Defibrillator pads are applied to the chest and a small jolt of electrical energy is delivered to the chest wall, which in most cases converts the AF to a normal sinus rhythm. These patients should be on blood thinners in advance to prevent any clot from getting to the brain.

Interventional treatment: People with chronic AF, and who have significant symptoms despite being on several medicines, may be candidates for radiofrequency ablation for AF. In the cardiac catheterization lab, multiple catheters are introduced from the groin vein and threaded up to the left upper chamber. The electrical activity of the atrium is monitored and certain areas, especially those surrounding the vein that drains into the atrium, are treated with radio-frequency waves, freezing and interrupting the abnormal electrical connections, thus stopping the AF. In experienced hands, it has a 70% success rate. These patients still need to maintain some medical regimen to reduce recurrences.

Pacemakers: Some people with AF who have very slow ventricular rates may not be able to maintain adequate blood circulation. These people may need a pacemaker to address a slow heart rate, and medicines to suppress a fast heart rate. Generally, a pacemaker procedure is performed in the cardiac catheterization lab. It is a fairly simple procedure where a wire is introduced via a shoulder vein into the right ventricle. A battery, which weighs less than an ounce, is connected to the wire. The battery stays underneath the skin.

Surgical procedure: When patients with coronary artery disease and AF go for bypass surgery, the surgeon may make an incision along the length of the atrial wall to disrupt any abnormal electrical connections in order to prevent AF.

Prognosis: AF is generally well controlled with medicines and is a well-tolerated rhythm problem. The risk of blood clot formation must be addressed to prevent stroke and loss of limb function.

Pacemakers

Ten years ago, Mr. Slone, a 68-year-old male, felt dizzy while driving. He pulled off the road and called for help. When he had arrived at the emergency room, his heart rate was in the low thirties. He underwent a permanent pacemaker insertion. For the next 9 to 10 years, his heart was solely dependent on the pacemaker to generate and maintain his heart rhythm at a steady rate of 75 beats per minute. Recently, he underwent a pacemaker battery replacement.

What maintains the cardiac rhythm? The heart is a muscular pump. Its rhythm is controlled by specialized groups of cells that have an inherent property to generate an impulse.

One such specialized group of cells located at the top of the right atrium is called the sinus node. The other group, where the upper and lower chambers join, is called the AV node. The impulse generated by these nodes is transmitted via a specialized network of heart muscle fibers called bundles. The sinus node beats at a rate of 60 to 100 times per minute, while the AV node can generate an impulse at a rate from 40 to 60 per minute. When both nodes fail, the heart muscle itself has the ability to generate an impulse, but it is too slow to maintain adequate cardiac function.

Rhythm problems: The most common rhythm problems that require pacemakers are slow heart rates resulting from sick sinus syndrome, AF with slow ventricular rates, and electrical blocks in the AV node.

Sick sinus syndrome is where the sinus node sometimes malfunctions with bursts of rapid rates mingled with very slow rates.

AF is a condition where the atria (upper chambers) beat at a rate of 350 to 400 beats per minute, while the ventricles beat at a much slower rate. Sometimes, the ventricular rate may be so slow that a pacemaker may be needed. AF is very common in people over 60. In patients who have both fast and slow heart rates due to AF, if we administer medicines to control the fast heartbeats, they may further aggravate the slow heart rhythm problem. Hence, a pacemaker will be necessary to address the slow heart rate, while medicines treat fast heartbeats.

When there is damage to the heart muscle, the tissue that transmits the electrical impulse (conduction system) may also get damaged, leading to electrical blocks in the AV node and very slow heart rates.

Types of pacemakers: During the dawn of the pacemaker era, maintaining a fixed rate was the main objective. However, the latest innovative technology has enabled us to use two or even three wires with a multitude of programming capabilities, including shocking (defibrillating) the heart if needed.

The most basic pacemaker has a battery and a pacemaker wire. The wire is placed in the right ventricle. This basically maintains the heart rhythm at a set rate and has some programming available to increase the rate if the demand goes up. This is useful in patients with chronic AF with very low heart rates.

The second type involves one wire in the left atrium (left upper chamber) and another wire in the right ventricle. Synchronizing the pacing of the atrium and the ventricle increases cardiac performance. This is helpful in patients with regular rhythm, stiff heart muscle, heart block, or congestive heart failure.

The third type involves placing three wires: one in the right upper chamber, one in the right ventricle, and a third one to pace the left ventricle in a synchronized manner. This technique simulates the normal heart contraction pattern and benefits patients with advanced heart failure and heart blocks by improving the pumping efficiency. Therefore, it is called cardiac resynchronization therapy (CRT).

The final type, the implantable cardioverter defibrillator (ICD), is able to shock the heart if it detects life-threatening arrhythmias. This also has full pacing capabilities. It has been shown to reduce death rates in patients with severely compromised heart function due to advanced heart failure with a pumping efficiency of less than 30% (a measure of efficiency called "Ejection Fraction or EF").

Diagnosis: A simple electrocardiogram may reveal a slow heart rate or a heart block. A 24-hour EKG monitoring device (Holter monitor) can pick up subtle slow heart rates and electrical blocks. An echocardiogram can reveal cardiac enlargement and advanced heart failure.

Pacemaker insertion: This procedure is routinely done in the cardiac catheterization laboratory under local anesthetic and light sedation.

After numbing the shoulder area with lidocaine, a needle is inserted in the main vein underneath the collar bone. A guide wire is passed through the needle. After establishing a venous access, a small incision is made in the skin, and an appropriately sized pocket underneath the skin is made for the pacemaker generator. A sheath is passed over the guide wire, through which one or two pacemaker wires are inserted. The wires are placed in the appropriate chambers under X-ray guidance. The pacemaker wires are tested to make sure they can sense the electrical impulse in the heart chamber and also pace adequately. The wires are attached to the generator and well secured. The generator is placed in the skin pocket and anchored with sutures. The skin is closed and a dressing applied. The patient is watched for 24 hours to make sure the pacemaker is functioning as intended. A chest X-ray is done to make sure there are no complications such as an air leak from the lungs or movements of the pacer wire.

Follow-up: Patients with pacemakers should be under the care of a qualified cardiologist. The pacemaker needs to be checked using a special machine that is specific to each brand of pacemaker. The pacemaker monitor will establish the proper functioning of the pacemaker and also helps to determine the battery life. From time to time, the pacemaker can be programmed to meet the current requirements.

Complications: Soon after the insertion of a pacemaker, the site must be kept clean to prevent any infection. The other problems associated with pacemaker insertion may include allergic reaction to the local anesthetic, bleeding, damage to a vein or an artery, and in rare cases, lung collapse.

Precautions: It is all right to use cell phones. However, you should avoid holding the cell phone too close to the pacemaker generator, as it may misinterpret the signal from the cell phone as a signal from the heart.

Passing through airport security may set off a metal detector, even though it may not interfere with the pacemaker function. Handheld devices should be kept away from the pacemaker. Always carry your pacemaker ID card with you.

Generally, microwave ovens, televisions, remote controls, radios, toasters, electric blankets, and electric shavers do not affect pacemakers. And yes, in 6 to 10 years, it may be time for a battery replacement.

Chapter 24

Medication Errors & Medicines That Don't Work

Medication Errors

Each year, medication errors account for more than 80,000 deaths and 770,000 injuries, at a cost of $2 billion and malpractice awards in excess of $660,000 for each serious outcome. It is a national health crisis that has gripped the attention of physicians, the public, and politicians.

Cases in point: A patient was prescribed 20 units of insulin. Instead, the patient receives 200 units, as 20 units was read as 200, resulting in the patent's death.

A patient develops severe bleeding from a commonly prescribed blood thinner, warfarin. The medicine was given four times a day instead of once daily, as the abbreviation qd (which stands for once daily) was misinterpreted as qid (which stands for four times daily). Here the error lies with the doctor, the pharmacist, and the nurse who administered the medicine. This error could have been detected at any level, if one person had used the knowledge that warfarin is given once daily and not four times a day.

A child is connected to a pain medicine pump after surgery for broken bones. In a rush, the nurse dials the adult dose for the morphine. In a few hours the child becomes very lethargic, gasping for air. If the mother had not woken up in the middle of the night, the child could have suffered serious damage from severe respiratory depression and hypotension.

Causes related to medication errors:

- Illegible prescriptions
- Transcription of orders
- Dispensing the wrong dose, frequency, or medicine
- Administering the wrong medicine by the nurse
- Selection of the wrong patient
- Failure to check for allergies
- Interaction with other medicines
- Stress
- Overwork
- Lack of communication
- Wrong route of administration (IV instead of oral)
- Failure to monitor side effects
- Distracting interruptions

Patients on diuretics (water pills) need close monitoring of electrolytes. Certain drugs are harmful to the kidneys (contrast agents used in diagnostic X-rays and CT scans, anti-inflammatory agents like Motrin, and others) and patients receiving such drugs need close observation of their kidney function. Patients with kidney failure also have trouble eliminating certain drugs, and therefore, the dosages of such drugs may have to be adjusted according to their kidney function. The same rule holds true for patients with liver or heart failure.

Drugs with very similar names:

- Serzone (nefazodone) for depression and Seroquel (quetiapine) for schizophrenia
- Lamictal (lamotrigine) for epilepsy, Lamisil (terbinafine) for nail infections
- Ludiomil (maprotiline) for depression, and Lomotil (diphenoxylate) for diarrhea
- Taxotere (docetaxel) and Taxol (paclitaxel), both for chemotherapy

- Zantac (ranitidine) for heartburn, Zyrtec (cetirizine) for allergies, and Zyprexa (olanzapine) for mental conditions
- Celebrex (celecoxib) for arthritis and Celexa (citalopram) for depression

Prevention Is Better Than Cure

Medication errors are multi-factorial and they involve a multi-disciplinary approach to recognize the problem and institute steps to prevent any further occurrences. We will look at the role of several players who are potentially involved in medication errors in preventing such mistakes.

Hospital's role: Most hospitals are taking aggressive proactive steps to eliminate certain abbreviations such as qd, qid, od, hs, and others. They are requiring doctors to spell out dosages and frequencies to avoid confusion. For example, thyroid hormones may be prescribed 100 mcg (microgram) or as 0.01 mg. Hospitals are incorporating very sophisticated software to detect any drug interactions and incompatibilities based on patient allergies.

Pharmacist's role: Pharmacists do intercept most medication errors. One study reported that 66% of the errors were detected by pharmacists. Yet, they cannot prevent all the medication errors, since the errors can occur long after the medicines leave the pharmacy department.

Physician's role: Generally, physicians are not very receptive to any behavior modifications in writing legible prescriptions, unless they have been a victim of a malpractice suit resulting from such errors. If you are getting an unusual number of calls from the pharmacy for clarification of your prescriptions, then it is time to have your prescriptions on the computer so you can print them instead of hand writing them. By doing so, you have a copy, the patient gets a copy, and the pharmacy calls are reduced in number.

Your role in medication error prevention: Make a list of all the diagnoses that apply to you.

Make a note of every medicine you are receiving in the hospital or from several doctors that you visit.

Include all the supplements and over-the-counter medicines that you take regularly and on occasion.

Chart the reasons for which your medicines are prescribed including the correct name, the dosage, the frequency, and the generic equivalents.

Make sure that your drugs match with your underlying medical condition(s). If they do not, don't accept that medicine until your physician explains why you need it. Make a note of that reason.

Check with the nurse or a pharmacist every time you receive a new medicine or unusual medicine.

Keep track of all your allergies, as any new medicine you receive may interact with existing medicines and result in an adverse reaction.

Be aware of similar sounding names and pills that may look alike, and that may be mistakenly dispensed because of a doctor's illegible handwriting.

Each time you visit your doctor, take all your medicines with you or have a complete list of all your medicines.

If you are on many medicines, put your daily medicines in a weekly prescription planner box (available at drug stores). This reduces the chances of an overdose or missed dose.

When Medicines Do Not Work

From time to time, my patients with hypertension or heart failure come back with worsening symptoms. When they do, I begin to wonder why the medicines that had done well before are unable to manage the disease or the symptoms now. Every practitioner faces a similar situation from time to time, whether he or she is dealing with a patient with bronchitis or severe diabetes.

The circumstances leading to a disparity between what a medicine is expected to do and what the outcome is could be related to the physician, the patient, the medicine itself, the circumstances, or a combination of factors.

Physician factors: A physician may have missed the diagnosis. It is not uncommon in a busy practice for a physician to overlook a symptom, especially when patients present with multiple health problems. Therefore, it is very important for the patient to make a list of the problems or concerns and seek answers to each of them from the physician or the physician's assistant. It is also important to give your physician a list of all the medicines that you are taking from several medical consultants that you are seeing on a regular basis.

It is also the responsibility of the physician to educate patients about the disease process and the importance of taking medicines for not only controlling symptoms, but also for preventing any possible complications. This is especially true when it comes to chronic illnesses such as hypertension, diabetes, arthritis, or heart disease. Your physician should provide proper diet information and other instructions that patients are expected to follow. That should help to alleviate the symptoms and accelerate the recovery from an acute illness. Controlling salt intake in case of hypertension, calories in case of diabetes, or water intake in heart failure are as essential as the medicines that are used to control these diseases. These points need to be reinforced to assure the patients understand and follow the instructions.

Patients must also be provided with written guidelines to follow so their efforts will complement the medicines' effects. Hospitals and emergency centers provide full written instructions for patients to follow besides taking their medicines properly or looking for symptoms that might signal worsening of the condition.

Doctors' handwriting has come under attack for patients getting the wrong medicine or the wrong dosage. The hospitals and the American Medical Association are taking a very proactive step in eliminating the misleading abbreviations and encouraging doctors to improve their handwriting or use computer generated prescriptions to minimize errors.

Medicines: Most medicines are first tested on laboratory animals and then a small segment of the population before they are approved by the U.S. Food and Drug Administration (FDA). That does not mean the drug would have the same intended effect on millions of people when it is released to the public. Take, for example, aspirin, a weak antiplatelet agent that is thought to reduce cardiovascular events by 25%. Most adults take an aspirin daily to prevent symptoms of heart disease.

However, more recent studies have shown that as many as 35% to 40% of people are so-called non-responders, meaning they do not get the needed antiplatelet effect to reduce cardiovascular events. Similar findings have been noted with Plavix, a stronger antiplatelet agent that is taken by patients who have received coronary stents. These patients may be at an increased risk of developing coronary thrombosis or blood clots. The reduced effectiveness may be addressed by increasing the dose to twice daily from a once-a-day dosage. A similar situation may exist when we are dealing with hypertension, where one or two medicines may not control blood pressure, thus forcing us to use three or even four different classes of drugs to control it. Similarly, blood sugar may not be well controlled when diabetes patients indiscriminately violate their diet instructions.

A combination of medicines may create an interaction, where one medicine may alter the effect of another medicine. So, when you see multiple doctors, it is very important to compile a list of all medicines so your doctors have a composite list of your medicines. When multiple blood pressure medicines are used, there is a tendency for salt retention, and you may need a stronger water pill to counteract that.

The disease process: Chronic illnesses are progressive. As the disease process evolves over years, the symptoms and the drug requirements may escalate. A clear understanding of this point will reinforce the importance of taking medicines regularly. You should take your medicines, even when you are not having any symptoms, to decrease the rate at which the disease progresses or leads to target organ damage, especially if you have diabetes and hypertension. It has been proven in multiple studies that reducing the risk factors for heart disease, such as cholesterol, decreases the rate of heart disease progression.

Patients with heart failure may develop fluid retention in the gut, which may interfere with absorption of medicines prescribed for that very condition, and their symptoms may get worse. Indiscriminate salt intake may make blood pressure medicines less effective.

Continued smoking may make medicines prescribed for bronchitis less effective, and as a result, the condition could get worse. Medicines given for heart failure may not work in the same manner in patients with abnormal kidney function versus those with normal kidney function. Heart failure itself can lead to worsening of kidney function, and therefore, close supervision may enable your doctor to adjust your medicine dosage, change, or add more drugs to get the desired effects.

The patient: I saved this section for last, so I can underscore the importance of you working in partnership with your physician to get the maximum benefit from the medicines that you take. When people are admitted to the hospital with a new onset of disease and their doctor prescribes medicine, they take it for some time. When they run out of the prescription, they feel they do not need that medicine anymore. Patients may be reluctant to take medicines because of lack of education on the importance of taking the medicines when they do not have symptoms.

The majority of the instances where medicines do not work as they are intended to are related to patients' failure to follow physician instructions or those provided by the pharmacist along with the prescriptions:

- Did you watch your diet?
- Did you quit smoking?
- Did you exercise?
- Did you lose weight?
- Did you take your medicines regularly?
- Did you follow up with your physician regularly?
- Do you understand the nature of your disease?
- Do you need a different drug?
- Do you need a different doctor?
- Are the medicines too expensive and can you get a generic version?

To get the maximum benefit from a given drug, first, the diagnosis has to be right. Next, the medicine prescribed must be the suitable drug of choice with minimal side effects and in the right dosage for the situation. Then, you need to follow the physician's instructions about what to do and what not to do, and be aware that chronic illnesses are progressive and need constant supervision.

When you follow these guidelines, and when the medicine fails to meet the intended purpose, then ask: Is it the doctor? Is it the patient? Is it the drug? Is it the disease process? Or is it a combination of factors?

Chapter 25

Women & Heart Disease

Heart Disease in Women

Heart disease is the leading cause of death among women. According to the Centers for Disease Control, it accounted for 27% of all deaths in the year 2004 in the United States. Nearly 500,000 women have heart attacks each year.

How are women different? Younger women have a lower incidence of heart disease compared with men. This is because of hormonal protection against arterial blockage and high HDL cholesterol levels. However, after menopause, the incidence of heart disease among women is equal to that seen in men. Thirty percent of women are likely to die in the first year following a heart attack in comparison to 25% of men.

Women have smaller coronary arteries. As a result, women are twice as likely as men to have complications following cardiac surgery. Women have a microvascular disease that involves very tiny arteries that are less suitable for angioplasty or bypass. Nonetheless, these small blocked arteries cause chest pain and shortness of breath. The treatment would include modification of risk factors to minimize the blockages in these small arteries.

Birth control pills can increase the risk of heart disease and stroke, especially in women with high blood pressure, diabetes and other risk factors.

There is a lack of relative knowledge among physicians regarding the magnitude and the seriousness of heart disease among women. Hence, women are often undertreated.

History: Most women do not present with the classic exertion-related chest pain. There is also a tendency in the medical field to attribute their symptoms to gastrointestinal problems such as gallstones, peptic ulcer, or stress. However, as an educated consumer, you want to ask your doctor to evaluate you for the heart disease risk factors and recommend tests to rule out heart disease.

Risk factors: The risk factors are cholesterol, diabetes, smoking, overweight, hypertension, and sedentary lifestyle.

Cholesterol: Cholesterol is the number one risk factor for heart disease in both men and women. The total cholesterol should be less than 200 mg% or less than 160 mg% in patients with diabetes. The LDL or the bad cholesterol must be close to 70 mg% to 80 mg%. The HDL or the good cholesterol is usually high in younger women. It should be more than 40 mg%.

Triglycerides: Elevated triglycerides (a type of fat in the blood) are an independent risk factor for heart disease among women. Elevated triglycerides are commonly seen in association with diabetes. When diabetes is controlled, the triglyceride levels come down. Other conditions that lead to elevated triglycerides would include excess carbohydrate or fatty diets, and alcohol.

Smoking: Smoking doubles the risk of heart disease. The risk of heart disease drops by a half, after one year of quitting smoking.

Blood pressure: The normal blood pressure is 120/80 mmHg. You can reduce your blood pressure with salt restriction, weight control, and exercise before you need any medicines.

Being overweight: Excess weight also can increase the risk of heart disease. It increases the risk of high blood pressure, diabetes, elevated cholesterol, and triglyceride levels. Weight control reduces most of the abovementioned risk factors. Keep your BMI below 25.

Diabetes: This disease is a very strong risk factor for heart disease. Strict control of diabetes can delay the rate at which most complications progress, including the development of heart disease symptoms.

Diagnostic Studies: Many diagnostic studies are available for the early detection of heart disease.

Electrocardiograms: They are of limited value in accurately diagnosing heart disease. Even the regular treadmill stress test is not very helpful in excluding heart disease, since 50% of the results can be false positives.

Nuclear stress test: It is more accurate in the diagnosis of heart disease. It also has limitations. Most women may not be able to reach the desired target heart rate during exercise. Additionally, the shadows cast by the breast may create artifacts interfering with the proper interpretation of the scans.

Positron emission tomography (PET): It may be useful in detecting microvascular disease.

CT angiography: This noninvasive study can detect coronary artery disease with a 98% specificity. That means, if the CT angiography is normal, the chance of having significant coronary artery disease is less than 2%.

Cardiac catheterization: It is considered the gold standard in the diagnosis of coronary artery disease. It is usually reserved as the last approach.

Treatment: The American Heart Association recommends that women with heart disease should receive aspirin (165 mg), beta blockers, and ACE inhibitors, in addition to cholesterol lowering drugs, multivitamins, and mineral therapy.

Hormone therapy: The role of hormone therapy has undergone several revelations. According to the latest studies, it has not been shown to reduce the incidence of heart disease. If hormones are primarily used for control of postmenopausal symptoms, your physician may consider a lower dose hormone for the shortest possible duration. Routine use of folic acid has not been shown to reduce the incidence of cardiovascular events.

Pregnancy & Heart Disease

From the time of the conception of a dream child to the realization of a newborn baby, the mother's cardiovascular system undergoes phenomenal changes. Some of these changes are a normal response to the excess demand created by the pregnancy, while a few others deserve closer attention.

Physiological changes during pregnancy: The mother's cardiovascular system experiences increased demand from the growing fetus, which begins around weeks 6 to 8 of pregnancy.

The cardiac output (the volume of blood put out by the heart each minute) increases by 40% to 50% and reaches a peak towards the end of the second trimester. This increase in cardiac output is due to an increase in blood volume, the amount of blood pumped during each heartbeat, and a slight increase in heart rate (10 to 15 beats per minute). There is a drop in blood pressure by about 10 mmHg due to dilation of the blood vessels.

Fluid retention during pregnancy is due to pressure on the large veins in the belly by the enlarging uterus. There may be a mild increase in heart size to accommodate the increased blood volume. Slight leg edema (swelling) may be noted.

During active labor, there is a displacement of almost 500 ml or one pint of blood from the uterus into the circulation, which increases the cardiac output. The blood pressure may rise in response to pain and anxiety.

Immediately following the delivery, there is an increase in venous blood return to the heart and subsequent increased cardiac output, which leads to a rapid increase in urine production. Most changes should be reversible in 1 to 2 weeks.

Cardiovascular symptoms of pregnancy: The abovementioned changes in the cardiovascular system can cause certain symptoms that are normal.

Due to increased intravascular blood volume and increased cardiac output, it is not uncommon to hear a heart murmur. The anemia associated with pregnancy dilutes the blood and may also contribute to a heart murmur. Some may also experience palpitations and irregular beats. The other symptoms may include shortness of breath, fatigue, and decreased exercise capacity. Some women may notice purple fingers due to reduced oxygen levels combined with poor circulation to the fingers. Other symptoms may include dizziness and occasional fainting, especially if the mother is dehydrated.

Pre-existing heart diseases: Patients with pre-existing cardiovascular problems such as rheumatic heart disease, heart failure and others must have prior consultation with their gynecologists and cardiologists to assess the risks and benefits of going through the pregnancy. The cardiovascular factors contributing to an adverse outcome during pregnancy are history of heart failure or stroke, history of significant arrhythmias requiring medicines, reduced functional capacity at rest, critical valvular heart disease, and reduced left ventricular function.

Mitral valve prolapse: This is a common condition noted in young women. Some of them might be on a beta-blocker such as atenolol or metoprolol. Inderal is the only beta-blocker that has been found to be safe during pregnancy. You need to be under the supervision of a cardiac specialist if you have any heart problems.

Blood thinners: Women may be on blood thinners for a variety of reasons such as having an artificial heart valve, cardiac enlargement, or significant cardiac arrhythmias. Most of these patients are on an oral blood thinner called warfarin (coumadin). This drug needs to be avoided, as its effects on the embryo and the fetus are unknown. Most pregnant women who need blood thinners are maintained with subcutaneous heparin or low molecular weight heparin during the first two trimesters of pregnancy. In rare cases, we may be able to resume coumadin after the first trimester and continue until the middle of the third trimester. Heparin does not cross the placenta. However, there is a very small risk of developing low platelet count with heparin. That risk is lower with low molecular weight heparin.

Diagnostic tests: During pregnancy, most doctors would avoid doing X-rays or other tests that can potentially harm the fetus. However, a simple electrocardiogram can detect irregular heart rhythms. A 24-hour Holter monitor also can help unravel any cardiac rhythm disturbances. Cardiac ultrasound is similar to the ultrasound used to evaluate the fetus. It is generally harmless. It can enable us to evaluate the heart size, thickness, function, and the origin of new heart murmurs. Blood tests may be performed to detect diabetes, thyroid disorders, and electrolyte imbalances that may be contributing to the cardiovascular symptoms. Based on these simple harmless studies, most cardiovascular problems during pregnancy can be addressed.

Treatment of cardiac symptoms: Most cardiovascular symptoms are self-limiting and do not have serious underlying cardiovascular causes. Hydration is an important point to keep in mind. Electrolyte disturbance that may cause palpitations can be avoided by proper nutrition. Close monitoring of weight gain is important.

Patients with heart failure or irregular heart rhythms can be treated with digoxin. We should avoid drugs that are used to treat hypertension or heart failure, like ACE inhibitors or ARBs, as they can cause kidney damage.

Patients with atrial fibrillation with a rapid ventricular response may be treated with beta-blockers, calcium channel blockers, or digoxin. Pregnancy related hormones increase the tendency for the blood to clot. Therefore, these patients may also need blood thinners such as heparin or low molecular weight heparin during a period of arrhythmias.

Adverse effects of medicines: Medicines given to treat the mother may also cross the placental barrier and reach the fetal circulation. So we need to be aware of the effects of medicines taken by the mother on the fetus. For example, beta-blockers given to the mother can cross the placental barrier and cause a reduction in the fetal heart rate. Similarly, ACE inhibitors can cross the placenta and cause fetal kidney tissue damage.

Preeclampsia: This is an abnormal condition associated with pregnancy. There is excess retention of fluids with elevated blood pressure and protein in the urine. If unrecognized and untreated in a timely manner, it could lead to seizure. There is slowing of fetal growth and an increased chance of early placental detachment. When the blood pressure goes over 150/100 mmHg, treatment with medicines is needed to keep the blood pressure under control and preserve kidney function.

Postpartum cardiomyopathy: This is a rare condition where the mother develops cardiac enlargement and obvious symptoms of heart failure associated with shortness of breath, leg swelling, and fatigue (1 in 3000 pregnancies). Some women may also complain of bloating and abdominal swelling. These symptoms can develop during the last weeks of pregnancy and continue for up to nine months after pregnancy. This is more commonly seen in women over age 30, with multiple pregnancies, and with a history of preeclampsia.

The treatment may include digoxin, diuretics, hydralazine, and beta-blockers. ACE inhibitors must be avoided to protect the kidneys. Patients with severe congestive heart failure may need anticoagulation treatment. The majority of the women recover normal heart function within 6 months after the onset of symptoms.

Diet & Heart Healthy Lifestyle for Women

- Keep calorie intake to 1200 to 1500 calories. Cut carbs.
- Reduce fat intake to less than 30% of total calories.
- Keep saturated fat intake to less than 10% of total calories.
- Consider Lean meat, less than 8 ounces per day.
- Exercise 20 to 30 minutes, 3 to 4 times per week.
- Use skim milk and vegetables.
- Consider oils rich in omega-3, such as fish oil or flax seeds/ oil supplements.
- Eat fish such as salmon, mackerel, or tuna, 2 to 3 servings per week.
- Drink a glass or red wine per day.
- Watch a comedy channel.
- Quit smoking.
- Drink 8 glasses of water/day.
- Eat grilled meat in place of meat with gravies.
- Take niacin 500 to 1000 mg/day.
- Avoid egg yolk, organ meat, solid fats, and canned foods.
- Keep salt intake less than 1 tsp/day.

Osteoporosis

What is osteoporosis? The bone is a spongy structure with a dense inner and outer covering. In osteoporosis, there is a decrease in bone mineral density, disruption of the microarchitecture, and increased bone fragility. Even though it is primarily a disease seen in postmenopausal women, it is also seen in men and in patients with chronic illness, and those who are on long-term steroids.

Risk factors: The most important risk factors are advanced age and the hormonal changes associated with that, namely reduced estrogen levels in females and reduced testosterone to a lesser degree in men. Other causes include chronic alcohol excess, vitamin D deficiency, smoking, lean body mass, lack of calcium in the diet, lack of exercise, exposure to cadmium, and possibly soft drinks containing phosphoric acid.

Mechanism of osteoporosis: There is continuous resorption of old bony material (removal of bony structures) and deposition of new bony matter in the body. This process is known as bone turnover or remodeling. A complete cycle of bone turnover or remodeling takes two to three months. The more bone mass you accumulate between the ages of 25 and 35, the less the risk of osteoporosis in the future.

Lack of estrogen leads to increased bone resorption. Calcium and phosphorus metabolism also plays a significant role in the removal and formation of bone. The parathyroid gland, located in the pituitary gland, at the base of the skull, controls the metabolism of calcium and phosphorus. When there is decreased calcium in the blood, the parathyroid gland stimulates the production of parathyroid hormone (PTH), which increases the bone resorption to maintain the blood calcium level. Other conditions that lead to osteoporosis include arthritis and kidney failure.

Complications: The most common complications are fractures or broken bones, which frequently occur in the wrist, spine, and hip. Collapsed vertebrae can cause severe and chronic back pain. Loss of height due to compression of the vertebrae can result in a stooping posture. Hip fractures are common in elderly people and can limit their activities. Hip surgery has its own complications.

Diagnostic tests: Very simple tests are available to screen people for early detection of osteoporosis. They measure the bone density. The best screening test is called dual energy X-ray absorptionmetry (DEXA). This test is simple, quick, and measures the bone density in the wrist, hip, and spine. This test is also useful in determining progress after implementing proper treatments. The bone density of a given patient is compared to that of a young adult used as a control. The results are interpreted as T-scores. A T-score of 1.0 is normal. When the results are between -1.0 and -2.5, the person is presumed to have an osteopenia or mild bone mass loss. A T-score of -2.5 or greater is indicative of osteoporosis. These criteria are useful in postmenopausal women and in men over the age of 50. A Z-score or comparison with age group rather than peak bone mass may also be necessary. Other tests include ultrasound and CT scans.

People over the age of 65, postmenopausal women, patients with history of fracture involving the weight-bearing bones, vertebral abnormalities, and those who are on long-term steroids for other conditions need screening. Other patients who need screening include those with diabetes, kidney failure, or early menopause. Screening is generally not recommended for younger men.

Drug treatment: Hormone replacement therapy is the primary approach to prevent further bone loss and perhaps increase the bone density. Estrogens alone or in combination with other agents are used in postmenopausal women. However, the hormones may have their own side effects, and you may have to consult with your gynecologist to determine the right hormone replacement in your situation.

Biphosphonates inhibit bone breakdown, preserve bone mass, and may even increase bone density. They may be especially useful in young men and those who are on long-term steroids. These drugs can be taken daily, weekly, or even once a month. Those who cannot tolerate the oral form may choose the intravenous route. Zoledronic acid (Reclast) is a new drug that can be given once a year intravenously in a doctor's office. It usually takes 15 minutes.

Raloxifene. It acts like the estrogen hormones without some of the risks associated with them, such as uterine or breast cancer. Women with a history of blood clots should not use this medicine.

Calcitonin, a hormone produced by the thyroid gland, reduces bone resorption, prevents spinal fracture, and reduces pain. It is given as a nasal spray. It is used in patients who cannot take biphosphonates.

Teriparatide (Forteo) is similar to PTH. It is one of the few agents that stimulate new bone formation. Like insulin, it has to be given subcutaneously (injected under the skin) once a day. It is still under investigation.

Tomoxifen, a synthetic estrogen hormone that is used in the treatment of breast cancer, has been shown to reduce bone resorption and reduce the risk of osteoporosis and fractures.

Prevention: Osteoporosis prevention is an important part of management of postmenopausal women.

Postmenopausal women should take at least 1000 mg of calcium and 800 units of vitamin D. Women who are at increased risk of osteoporosis should take 1500 mg of calcium per day. Food sources, such as milk, broccoli, almonds, canned salmon with the bones, oats, and tofu are good sources of calcium. Constipation related to calcium can be counteracted by increased water and fiber intake.

Exercise definitely helps to strengthen your muscles and increase your bone density. It is best to start at an early age when your body is still building your bones. Weight-bearing exercises such as walking, running, stair climbing, or rope jumping can help to strengthen the bones in the legs, hip, and back. Low-impact exercises done on an elliptical machine may provide cardiovascular benefits, but are less effective in increasing bone strength.

Soy products are known to contain plant estrogens, which may be beneficial in patients with osteoporosis. Smoking reduces estrogen levels, increases bone resorption, and interferes with calcium absorption in the gut. Limit your caffeine intake to less than 2 to 3 cups of coffee per day.

Maintain a good body posture while standing and sitting at your desk all day long. When you are sitting, use a rolled towel or a pillow to support your lower back. Make sure your back is supported when you lift, carry, or push heavy objects. Avoid falling by keeping the floor dry and using comfortable shoes.

Chapter 26

Hypertension & Hypotension
Either way, they spell trouble

Hypertension

More than 60 million people in America have hypertension. Hypertension is a silent killer, as it does not produce significant symptoms. However, it can cause serious organ damage from stroke, heart failure, heart attack, kidney failure, or arterial blockage in the legs. Less than one-third of the hypertensive people are well controlled on their treatment.

Why treat hypertension? Hypertension, if uncontrolled, can cause severe bleeding in the brain or a stroke. Adequate control of blood pressure can reduce the risk of stroke by 60%.

Longstanding hypertension is a leading cause of congestive heart failure. Good control of blood pressure can prevent the thickening and enlargement of the heart and reduce the risk of heart attacks that weaken the heart muscle.

Uncontrolled hypertension can eventually lead to kidney failure, necessitating dialysis in the long run.

The hypertension treatment cost is minimal, compared with that of managing any of the complications. Most hypertension can be controlled with one or two medicines. The cost of three months' supply could be less than you spend for an evening's dinner.

Lifestyle changes: The treatment of hypertension begins with you. Reducing your weight and engaging in regular exercise bring down your blood pressure. Alcohol, caffeine, and smoking temporarily increase blood pressure. Routine blood pressure checks help you to monitor your blood pressure and adjust your medications so your blood pressure is controlled throughout the day. Meditation and relaxation techniques that reduce stress can lower blood pressure.

Diet and salt restriction: There is a direct correlation between blood pressure and salt intake. Excess sodium in the blood vessel walls makes the walls stiff and raise their resistance to blood flow, and thus increase blood pressure. Some people are more sensitive to salt than others. Nonetheless, all patients with blood pressure problems must watch their salt intake. Reducing the salt intake can lower blood pressure. Replacing regular salt with salt substitutes can also help. Dash is a salt substitute that contains potassium instead of sodium. However, you need electrolyte monitoring to ensure that you are not getting excess potassium, especially in the presence of kidney disease. A diet low in calories and fat helps you to lose weight and reduce the cholesterol deposition in the arterial walls that increases the resistance to blood flow.

Water pills: Water pills or diuretics increase the removal of sodium in the urine, reduce the sodium content in the arterial walls, and decrease the resistance to blood flow, thus reducing blood pressure. Water pills also increase the removal of potassium, and therefore, some patients may need potassium supplements and routine electrolyte monitoring. There are potassium sparing diuretics (Maxzide, Aldactone) that conserve potassium. They may have a tendency to raise potassium levels too much if not closely monitored. You should also minimize sodium-rich foods such as pickles, soups, and tomato juice.

Beta-blockers: Beta-blockers reduce the heart rate and reduce blood pressure. The most common beta-blockers on the market are Inderal, atenolol, and metoprolol. Beta-blockers may increase bronchial spasm in patients with asthma or chronic lung disease, worsen the symptoms of arterial disease in the legs, and mask hypoglycemia (low blood sugar) symptoms. They reduce the risk of heart attack and sudden death. The slowed heart rate can be a problem with some patients.

ACE inhibitors: Angiotensin II converting enzyme (ACE) inhibitors are very potent agents that reduce the arterial wall tension and lower blood pressure. Therefore, it may be necessary to take water pills along with large doses of ACE inhibitors. The most commonly used ACE inhibitors are enalapril, Monopril, lisinopril, and quinapril. They are also useful in a variety of conditions such as heart failure, coronary artery disease, diabetes, kidney disease, and heart attack, among others. They may also cause a dry hacking cough and could become bothersome in patients with chronic lung disease. They also may increase potassium levels in patients who are on supplemental potassium with water pills. Occasionally, people may develop a rash, dizziness, or lightheadedness. The ACE inhibitors are the most widely prescribed group of medicines for hypertension. Women who plan on getting pregnant must avoid these drugs, as they can cause birth defects.

ARBs: ARBs are another class of drugs that have effects similar to ACE inhibitors, thus reducing the arterial wall tension and blood pressure.

The most commonly used ARBs are losartan (Cozaar), valsartan (Diovan), irbesartan (Avapro), and candesartan (Atacand).

They are as effective as the ACE inhibitors. Unlike ACE inhibitors, the ARBs do not produce dry cough. They increase salt and water retention, which can increase blood pressure. Other side effects may include headache and dizziness.

Calcium channel blockers: Calcium channel blockers (CCBs) block the entry of calcium into the heart muscle and blood vessel walls, which reduces resistance and blood pressure.

The most commonly used CCBs are diltiazem, nifedipine, verapamil, and amlodipine.

Verapamil can slow the heart rate and reduce the heart's pumping function, and should be used with caution in heart failure patients.

Nifedipine can increase heart rate and oxygen needs of the heart. Its short-acting forms must be avoided in patients with heart disease, as they can cause a heart attack.

Cardizem has a tendency to slow the heart rate.

Other side effects include constipation, leg swelling and flushing.

Centrally acting agents: These drugs reduce the arterial wall resistance and blood pressure. The most commonly used agent is Clonidine. It has to be taken two to three times daily. The major side effects are drowsiness, fatigue, impotence, constipation, dry mouth, and weight gain. Abrupt stopping can cause a recurrence of high blood pressure.

Vasodilators: They dilate the blood vessels and reduce blood pressure. Hydralazine and minoxidil are commonly used vasodilators. Minoxidil can drop blood pressure too much in a standing position. These are used as the last resort for hypertension treatment. Hydralazine can increase the chance of developing lupus, an autoimmune disease.

Combination drugs: Generally, I avoid using combination drugs, since it is difficult to adjust the dosages. When the blood pressure is moderate or severe, we need to use two or more medicines to get the desired effect. When you are on more than two medicines for blood pressure control, make sure you are taking a water pill to reduce salt retention.

Hypotension

Nancy, a young lawyer in her early thirties, came to my office with her sister for a check-up.

I said, "You do not look like one of my regular patients. What brings you to our office?"

"My sister. She thinks I need to see a cardiologist!"

"Do you have any problems?"

"Besides my sister? I feel weak and dizzy in the morning hours. I feel tired all the time."

"When is the last time you had a medical checkup?"

"Every day! My sister has done all types of blood work and tests. However, she cannot figure it out."

"She always runs low blood pressure," said Nancy's sister, a physician.

"Well, Nancy, what is your height and weight?" I asked.

"I am 5 feet 4 inches tall. I weigh 110 pounds. I'm active."

"What time do you go to work?"

"I leave home at 7:00 a.m."

"Do you get coffee or breakfast?"

"I never have breakfast."

"Did your sister check you for diabetes?"

"Oh, yes! I passed a five hour glucose test."

"Do you experience palpitations?"

"Ah, yes! When I stand up, for no reason, my heart speeds up, and then I feel dizzy."

"What else?" I said.

"I have no energy. I could have two energy drinks, and I still feel like I have no energy. Sometimes I feel like I'm ready to faint. At times, my hands and feet feel cold and look pale. Occasionally, my vision gets blurred."

"Well, let me check your blood pressure."

I checked her blood pressure while she was lying down and standing. I said, "Your blood pressure while lying was 96/60 and while standing it was 88/60 mm Hg."

"What does that mean?"

"You run low blood pressure."

"What causes low blood pressure?"

"Several conditions can cause low blood pressure in young people. Dehydration is a common cause. People who are taking weight control pills may inadvertently be getting water pills that can make them get dehydrated, leading to low blood pressure."

"Do I look like someone who needs weight control pills?"

"Then we can eliminate that as the cause."

"All right," Nancy said.

"Dizziness can be caused by a number of things and low blood sugar is certainly something to consider. Since you already had a glucose test, we can exclude that as the cause of your dizziness."

"Then why do I have low blood pressure?"

"In some young people, the cause of low blood pressure is unknown. Normally, after prolonged standing, the brain receives signals that there is pooling of blood in the legs. However, in some people with brain chemical imbalance, the brain receives a signal from the heart that the blood pressure is indeed high and thus sends signals to further lower the blood pressure, which can lead to dizziness and fainting."

"That is interesting!" Nancy said.

"Young people with low body mass may have low blood pressure. A number of things that you are doing are not helping the situation."

"Such as?" Nancy asked.

"Not maintaining adequate hydration."

"How?" Nancy quizzed.

"Look at your history. You do not eat anything all night and do not have any breakfast. At the same time, your body is losing fluids through metabolism, sweating, and in the urine. When you are losing fluids, you lose water and salt. But when you replace fluids, you drink plain water or soft drinks. They do not replenish the salt that holds water in the blood vessels."

"Is this another way of saying that I need to eat something before I go to work?"

"Well, hydration is the key to maintain intravascular volume. You have seen football players walking around with Gatorade bottles and not water bottles. You may consider drinking skim milk or having a good breakfast in the morning."

"What if the symptoms do not get better?"

"Some patients may have what we call a poor vasomotor tone."

"Meaning?"

"Their blood vessels cannot maintain steady vascular tone which can quickly adjust to changes in fluid volume, hormonal variations, or posture."

"What do you do then?"

"Wearing elastic stockings can prevent the blood from pooling, especially when you stand up suddenly. Before you change your posture from lying or sitting to a standing position, you may dangle your feet a few times to pump the blood back to the heart.

"What if that doesn't work?"

"Also we recommend people to take salt tablets. Yes, I know. It does not taste like chocolate. But it feels better than dizziness and tiredness. Soup or tomato juice with high sodium content also can help. Pickles are also high in salt and help to maintain blood pressure. Avoiding heavy meals will also reduce the shifting of the blood to the gut from the main circulation. "

"If that doesn't work?"

"We consider some drugs."

"I don't want to take any pills." Nancy was determined.

"That is why I suggested some simple measures such as maintaining hydration, using elastic stockings, changing posture with caution, avoiding prolonged exposure to hot weather, and increasing your salt intake."

"What pills are you talking about?"

"These are known as alpha stimulants like midodrine that increase blood vessels' smooth muscle tone and increase the vascular tone to maintain effective intravascular volume. Fludrocortisone increases the salt retention in the body and blood volume."

"Oh, hold it! I wasn't looking for such an elaborate technical description," Nancy said. Then she turned to her sister and said, "Did you understand what he said?"

"Just be quiet and pay attention," replied her sister.

Three months later, I saw Nancy at a social gathering. I said, "Hi, Nancy."

She said, "I'm fine. I'm eating breakfast, drinking soup, avoiding heat, and carrying salt tablets. I don't think I need those pills now. Bye!"

Notes:

Chapter 27

Diabetes & Thyroid Problems

Diabetes & Heart Disease

Heart disease and diabetes are very common in the adult population. One disease complicates the other. Diabetes is a major risk factor for heart disease and increases illness and death in heart patients.

Special cardiac concerns: The cardiovascular risks and outcomes in a newly diagnosed diabetic patient are equal to those of a non-diabetic patient with a heart attack. More than 75% of the deaths in diabetics are related to cardiovascular system (CVS) complications. Diabetics have twice the risk of developing heart disease, in comparison to those without diabetes. They develop these complications at an earlier age and die prematurely. The incidence of heart disease among diabetic women has been on the rise in the past few decades.

Accelerated atherosclerosis: Diabetes is more than just blood sugar control. It is a systemic disease which has a multitude of complications, including elevated lipid levels, changes in small and medium size arteries, and changes in the heart, kidneys, and brain, thus affecting many target organs. The high blood sugar is harmful to the inner lining of the blood vessels (endothelium), which leads to overgrowth of smooth muscles in the arterial wall, in turn leading to increased atherosclerosis (narrowing of arteries). Diabetics also have a higher tendency to form blood clots (increased thrombogenicity).

In addition, diabetic patients very often have high blood pressure, elevated and abnormal cholesterol, triglycerides, and inflammatory markers such as C-reactive protein (CRP). They have smaller, denser, more oxidized LDL (bad cholesterol), which is very harmful to the arterial walls. The HDL cholesterol levels are generally lower among diabetics.

All these factors increase the CVS risks. Fortunately, many of these risk factors can be modified with diet and proper treatment, thus reducing the long-term complications.

Metabolic syndrome: Some people may not meet all the criteria for full-blown diabetes, but may have several abnormalities that increase their CVS risk. One such condition is called "metabolic syndrome," which is defined by the presence of obesity (belt size > 40" in men and > 35" in women); triglycerides > 150 mg%, HDL < 40 mg% in men and <50 mg% in women; blood pressure >130/85 mm Hg; and a fasting blood sugar >100 mg%. People who have three or more of these factors must seek medical attention to begin an aggressive treatment plan to minimize, or at least delay, future complications.

Coronary interventions: Diabetics have smaller coronary arteries with multiple plaque formations, in contrast to non-diabetics. They also have a higher incidence of totally blocked coronary arteries. Patients receiving bare metal stents have a much higher incidence of developing scar tissue inside the stent. The drug eluding stents may decrease recurrence of blockage in the same area. Since diabetics have multiple blockages and diffuse disease, stents may not be a suitable choice in every patient. However, stents used in large vessels in strategic locations may postpone the need for urgent bypass surgery.

Heart surgery: If complete establishment of circulation is not attainable with stents, coronary artery bypass surgery may be the best option. Women with diabetes who go for heart surgery may have more complications compared with men. The incidence of chest wound infection in diabetics is higher in comparison to that in non-diabetics. Strict blood sugar control may reduce the incidence of infection following surgery. Recovery following surgery is prolonged because of multiple factors such as infection, poor blood sugar control, obesity, and kidney problems. Patients who have bypass surgery seem to have fewer cardiac symptoms after surgery in comparison to those who are treated with stents. There is also evidence to suggest that the long-term survival rates in diabetics undergoing heart surgery are better compared to those who undergo coronary intervention.

Heart failure: Diabetics also have a higher incidence of heart failure due to uncontrolled high blood pressure, multiple heart attacks, small coronary arteries with generalized narrowing, kidney failure, and possible microvascular disease. Management of heart failure in diabetics is more challenging due to shifts in blood fluid volume due to high blood sugar level and associated kidney problems.

Peripheral arterial disease (PAD): PAD involves blockage of the arteries in the legs, leading to poor circulation and pain. This is covered in depth in the chapter on arterial diseases. The incidence of PAD is much higher in diabetics. It gets worse if the patient continues to smoke. Here also, patients have more generalized narrowing and more critical blockages. They do poorly with interventions such as balloon angioplasty or stents. Bypass surgery may temporarily help. It is extremely difficult to reestablish circulation in patients with severe blockages below the knee level. In the long run, poor circulation can lead to gangrene, forcing amputation. In fact, diabetes is the leading cause of leg amputations.

Stroke: People with diabetes are four times more likely to have a stroke in comparison to non-diabetics. Following a first stroke, the risk of a subsequent stroke increases two to four times.

Diabetes treatment: It is very important to understand the disease and take proper steps, including lifestyle modifications, diet adjustments, and exercise. Education is the key to success. Blood glucose varies constantly, related mostly to diet. Home glucose monitoring is extremely important. If you do not check, you do not know your glucose levels, and you cannot treat what you do not know.

Insulin or oral pills? This depends on the patient's need—the key is to maintain a reasonable target blood glucose range.

Certain pills have added CVS protection while others are neutral. Insulin is often needed to control blood glucose in longstanding or poorly controlled diabetes—it should not be seen as a "defeat." Both pills and insulin can cause low blood glucose or hypoglycemia, and that has some added risk in patients with CVS disease; therefore the need for monitoring and education to prevent such mishaps.

From the medical studies, it is evident that for each point drop in the HgA1c (a measure of long-term blood glucose control), there is a 13% reduction in cardiovascular disease. Similarly to cholesterol, there is a direct correlation between glucose control and the incidence of CVS complications. So, aggressive control of diabetes as well as other risk factors (like blood pressure and cholesterol) has a significant benefit in reducing deaths from CVS in the long run. The American Diabetes Association recommends bringing HgA1c levels to below 7.0% but others recommend below 6.5% (normal is 6%).

The steps necessary to minimize the deadly CVS complications of diabetes depend on a team approach between you and your physicians and addressing diet, blood sugar levels, blood pressure, cholesterol levels, exercise, and weight control.

In addition, you should consider the following measures:
- Education and knowledge
- Monitoring Blood sugar daily
- Controlling your weight
- Managing lipids
- Keeping LDL < 80 to 100 mg%
- Keeping HgA1c < 6 to 7%
- Reducing blood pressure to <130/80 mm Hg
- Exercising 20 to 30 minute 3 to 4 times weekly
- Avoiding infections and smoking
- Considering aspirin and Plavix
- Knowing that bypass surgery may be better than stents for patients with coronary artery disease.
- Considering ACE inhibitors to protect the kidneys

The American Diabetes Association has taken the initiative to promote the awareness of a link between diabetes and heart disease or stroke.

Visit:

www.americanheart.org/

www.diabetes.org/

and learn more about these and other conditions.

Thyroid Hormone & Heart Disease

An estimated 27 million Americans suffer from thyroid disease and half of them are undiagnosed or not treated. Women are seven times more likely to develop thyroid disease than men.

The thyroid gland is located in the neck, just below the Adam's apple. It produces a thyroid hormone called thyroxine that controls the body's metabolic rate. The thyroid gland itself is controlled by thyroid stimulating hormone (TSH) secreted by the pituitary gland, which is located at the base of the brain. The pituitary gland, responding to stimuli from the body and based on metabolic signals, triggers the thyroid gland to produce more thyroid hormone, and reduce the production of TSH.

Thyroid hormone: The thyroid gland produces many hormones, of which triiodothyronine (T3) and thyroxine (T4) are important. Thyroid hormone is delivered to the body's cells via the blood. At the cellular level, the hormone helps the cells to convert oxygen and calories into energy needed to sustain life and maintain metabolism.

Thyroid hormone controls the body's metabolism. Abnormalities of thyroid gland can lead to either high or low thyroid production, either of which can have an adverse effect. We encounter patients with both high and low thyroid hormone levels that have significant cardiac symptoms.

High-risk population: Patients with a family history of thyroid disease, autoimmune disease, fibromyalgia, recent pregnancy, menopause, smoking, exposure to radiation, and chronic fatigue syndrome are at increased risk of developing thyroid problems.

Hyperthyroidism: High levels of thyroid hormone are seen mostly in young adults between the ages of 25 and 50. Grave's disease is where the thyroid gland is affected by an autoimmune state that leads to enlargement and excess thyroid hormone formation. It affects about 5 in 10,000 people.

Excess thyroid hormone increases the body's metabolism. Patients may have anxiety, irritability, sleep disorders, excess sweating, changes in hair and skin, palpitations, shortness of breath, weight loss, heat sensitivity, visual disturbances and emotional problems.

Excess hormone also leads to increased work for the heart. Over a prolonged period, this excess load on the heart could lead to heart enlargement and heart failure. Hyperthyroidism patients also will exhibit other findings of thyroid disease such as an enlarged thyroid gland and bulging eyes.

Hypothyroidism: Low thyroid hormone levels are seen at all ages from the twenties and beyond. It can result from removal of the thyroid gland, inflammation, or radioactive treatment of a hyperactive thyroid gland, among other causes. An autoimmune disease called Hashimoto's disease causes inflammation of the thyroid gland. It is the most common cause of hypothyroidism in young people, especially women.

Hypothyroid patients may present with weakness, lethargy, lack of energy, sleepiness, weight gain, depression, swelling in the legs, constipation, loss of hair, intolerance to cold, and difficulty in concentrating or thinking. They also can develop heart failure and fluid around the heart. If untreated, it can lead to coma. The EKG may show decreased voltage. The chest X-ray may reveal a globe shaped heart due to enlargement and fluid collection.

Diagnosis: A simple blood test can measure both the thyroid hormones (T3 and T4) and TSH. It will enable establishing clear-cut cases of high or low thyroid hormone situations. Sometimes, borderline results may not reveal the low or ineffective thyroid state at the tissue level. Further testing has to be done to determine whether the tests really reflect the actual condition or the results are abnormal because of other hormonal changes in the body. A radioactive iodine uptake test is used to diagnose hyperthyroidism. Thyroid studies are also advisable during early pregnancy and in adults over the age of 50.

Other diagnostic tests include an ultrasound test to determine the presence of enlargement, nodules, and cysts. The nodules can be hot or cold depending on whether they are producing hormones or not. A fine-needle aspiration may reveal an unsuspected cancer of the thyroid gland.

Treatment: The treatment of low thyroid is much easier than the treatment of a high thyroid situation. When patients have low thyroid hormone, all they have to do is to replace the thyroid hormone with the drug levothyroxine or T4 (50 to 200 micrograms) until there is enough of it in the body. This can be established by measuring the TSH level. In a hypothyroid patient, the TSH levels are high. As the thyroid hormone is replaced, the TSH level gradually drops and reaches a normal range. Thus, the TSH serves as a guide to determine the optimal levothyroxine dose in each individual.

It is necessary to monitor cardiac symptoms while the thyroid hormone is being replaced. When the thyroid hormone is replaced aggressively, it can increase the demand on the heart and cause a new set of heart related symptoms. Too much thyroid hormone may also lead to bone loss. Therefore, periodic thyroid hormone measurement and adjustment of the thyroid hormone intake is essential. Most patients need to be on thyroid hormone replacement for the rest of their lives. Patients with heart disease must be started on a very low dose of thyroid hormone (25 to 50 micrograms) and the dose gradually increased, depending on the cardiac symptoms.

Hyperthyroidism treatment includes pills to suppress thyroid hormone production (methimazole and propylthiouracil) and beta-blockers to minimize the cardiovascular effects. Radiation and surgery may be needed, depending on the diagnosis. Total thyroid gland removal may be indicated when cancer is suspected.

It is important to recognize hyperthyroidism at its early stage to prevent permanent changes in the eyes and heart.

Bio-identical hormones may be sold as a superior form of hormone replacement. However, if your disease symptoms are controlled on synthetic hormones, then there is no need for a more expensive version. If your symptoms persist, then consult an endocrinologist.

Chapter 28

Congestive Heart Failure (CHF)

CHF Medical Management

It was 3 p.m. I got a call from the emergency center, about one of my patients, who was short of breath with a heart rate more than 160 beats per minute. An ultrasound test revealed a heart that was greatly enlarged, twice the normal size, barely moving with a heart function of 7 to 8% (normal 50 to 70%). It was baffling to see a 50-year-old man in this condition, being able to talk and comprehend. We brought his heart rate down. Thanks to modern medicine, three years later, he is fully employed with a heart function in the range of 40% to 43%. He is a classic textbook case of congestive heart failure (CHF), and how modern medicine can alter the course of events in patients with similar conditions.

What is CHF? The heart is a muscular organ which pumps 50% to 70% of the blood it receives with each heartbeat. When the heart muscle gets weak for various reasons, the pumping efficiency is reduced. So, more blood is left behind in the heart chamber with each heartbeat. That, combined with the weakness in the heart muscle itself, leads to enlargement of the heart chambers, eventual fluid retention, and the symptoms associated with CHF.

What causes CHF? The common causes of CHF are long-standing hypertension, coronary artery disease, diabetes, and valvular heart disease. In some patients, it may be related to a viral infection or alcohol excess. In all these cases, there is damage to the heart muscle, which weakens the pumping action of the heart. This leads to accumulation of salt and water, which further increases the heart's size, and the process continues until the heart chamber becomes very big with very thin and weak walls. This flabby heart cannot pump enough blood to the rest of the body. The reduced blood flow to the kidneys leads to retention of salt and water, which worsens the symptoms of CHF.

How do you diagnose CHF? As the heart muscle weakens, people experience shortness of breath with minimal exertion or even at rest. Due to reduced cardiac output, some people experience weakness, tiredness, and lack of energy. In addition, they may develop swelling in the legs and weight gain. If untreated, they could develop acute pulmonary edema, where their lungs get filled with fluid, making it difficult for the person to breathe. Some people may have lack of appetite and indigestion due to buildup of fluid in the gut. Rarely, people may have altered mental status due to reduced oxygen delivery to the brain.

Examination may reveal heart enlargement, lung congestion, and leg swelling. The electrocardiogram (EKG) may show evidence of old heart attacks or heart enlargement. The chest X-ray may show a big heart with lung congestion.

An ultrasound may reveal an enlarged heart with significantly reduced left ventricular function. The left ventricular pumping efficiency or the left ventricular ejection fraction (EF) is normally in the range of 50% to 70%. However, in patients with severe CHF, it may range from 10% to 30%.

Blood tests may reveal elevated brain natriuretic peptide (BNP) in chronic CHF. Computerized tomography (CT) and magnetic resonance imaging (MRI) also can detect the presence of an enlarged heart. Angiograms will help us to identify coronary artery disease.

How do we treat CHF? CHF management is a team effort between the physician and the patient. Patients should follow proper instructions to get the maximum benefit from leading-edge medical treatments that minimize the symptoms, improve the quality of life, and increase survival.

Digitalis: It has been used for more than 100 years for heart failure treatment. It strengthens the heart muscle, controls the heart rate, and helps to eliminate the buildup of salt and water. It works better in acute heart failure.

Diuretics: Drugs such as furosemide (Lasix) and HCTZ remove the extra salt and water from the body and thus reduce lung congestion and improve shortness of breath. At first, you may need a small dose. However, when the kidneys begin to fail, the diuretic dose may have to be increased. Diuretics have a tendency to waste potassium and therefore regular potassium monitoring and replacement may be needed.

Beta-blockers: Drugs such as atenolol, Lopressor and carvedilol slow the heart rate, reduce the work load on the heart, and improve survival. Carvedilol has been shown to improve symptoms and reduce hospital admission for CHF patients.

ACE inhibitors: ACE inhibitors are drugs that act to reduce levels of a set of hormones (the renin angiotensin system) that control blood pressure and fluid balance in patients with CHF. The ACE inhibitors reduce the strain on the heart muscle, reduce the heart size, improve the heart function, and prolong life.

Blood pressure control with other medicines, if needed, is essential. If a patient has severe triple-vessel coronary artery disease, bypass surgery could improve the symptoms of CHF.

Aldosterone antagonists: Drugs such as Aldactone and eplerenone (Inspra) have been shown to improve CHF symptoms, reduce the scarring of the heart muscle, and improve survival.

How to prevent CHF? We should control high blood pressure and reduce the risk factors for heart attack. Once there is damage to the heart muscle, it is permanent. We cannot repair that. Therefore, it is essential to minimize further damage by reducing the risk factors. Without proper treatment, the mortality rates for severe CHF patients used to be 50% over two years. However, with treatment, we can significantly improve their life expectancy.

What is the patient's role in CHF management? Patients should maintain strict weight control, minimize their salt (less than 2 grams per day) and water intake, take medicines regularly, and engage in moderate exercise. Regular medical checkups may reduce hospital admissions.

CHF Surgical Management

Patients with CHF also suffer from various other cardiac problems besides heart muscle weakness. Therefore, a variety of surgical options are available to improve their overall heart function and to prolong life in certain individuals.

Surgical procedures aimed at the heart rhythm could include pacemakers and defibrillators.

Pacemakers: Patients with advanced heart failure may develop abnormalities in cardiac rhythm such as atrial fibrillation, sick sinus syndrome, and heart blocks. Atrial fibrillations can seriously compromise the already failing heart function. Some patients may undergo a technique called radiofrequency ablation, to restore the normal sinus rhythm. This procedure is done in a cardiac catheterization laboratory, where several catheters are placed in the patient's heart to map the electrical activity of the heart. Certain areas in the heart muscle with an abnormal electrical activity are identified and frozen using catheters that deliver radio-frequency waves. This radio frequency ablation procedure is very effective in converting the atrial flutter arrhythmias to normal sinus rhythm in more than 95% of the patients. It also can convert atrial fibrillation to sinus rhythm in 70% of the patients.

Cardiac resynchronization therapy (CRT): More than 50% of patients may have heart rhythm and electrical conduction problems that can cause the left and right ventricles to contract out of sequence, thus reducing the overall heart efficiency. These people may benefit from a biventricular pacemaker that restores cardiac synchronization and improves the performance of heart function. Here, both the ventricles are made to contract at the same time by pacing both ventricles simultaneously.

Implantable cardiac defibrillators (ICDs): Ventricular arrhythmias may pose a serious hazard in patients with CHF, including rare cases of sudden death. Patients with reduced left ventricular pumping function (EF of less than 35%) are especially prone to such arrhythmias. These patients may benefit from ICDs. If a heart develops a seriously abnormal rhythm, such as a ventricular fibrillation, these devices shock the heart to restore the normal rhythm. ICDs are miniature versions of automatic defibrillator devices used on planes and in the hospital to shock people who are in cardiac arrest from ventricular fibrillation. However, since the device is inside the body and connected to the heart with a wire, the amount of energy released is very small. Nonetheless, when this device goes off, patients can a feel a small jolt coming from within the chest.

Valve replacement: Some patients may have a severe valve leak that can lead to heart failure. In such patients, replacement of the heart valve can prevent further deterioration in the heart function. There are two kinds of values, namely mechanical and bioprosthetic (valves made from tissue from cows or pigs). All patients receiving mechanical valves have to be on a blood thinner such as warfarin, which requires regular blood checks to monitor its effectiveness. Most patients who receive the bioprosthetic values may not need the blood thinner.

Aneurysm resection and bypass surgery: Some patients with a history of heart attack may develop thinning and stretching of the heart muscle to a point where it bulges outward instead of contracting with each heartbeat, thus reducing the pumping efficiency of the heart. If a patient is going for coronary artery bypass surgery to improve the circulation, the surgeon may also remove the scar tissue and reduce the left ventricular size to improve the heart function. People who have triple vessel coronary artery disease with heart failure do better after bypass compared with those treated with medicines alone.

Left ventricular assist device (LVAD): Patients with advanced heart failure, who can barely maintain blood circulation at rest, may need additional support to just sustain life. Such patients may benefit from an artificial pump called an LVAD that is attached to the tip of the left heart chamber. This device pumps the blood forward with each heartbeat. The modern devices can pump as much as 5 liters of blood per minute to sustain life. However, this is a temporary measure in patients with severe heart failure who are waiting for a donor heart transplant. Nonetheless, these devices have been left in place for months in some patients with reasonable success. Since LVADs are a foreign object, there is an increased risk of infection or blood clot formation.

Heart transplant: Younger people with severe heart failure who fail to respond to maximum medical treatment may be candidates for heart transplant. However, the transplant process cannot be taken lightly. It is a very intense process where all systems such as kidneys, lungs, liver, etc. are evaluated along with a psychological assessment and available social support, to determine the eligibility for heart transplant. This may take 18 to 24 months. In addition, patients should not have any debilitating diseases. When a donor heart becomes available, the recipient's left and right ventricles are removed, leaving only a part of the atria or the upper chambers. The donor's atria are joined to the recipient's atria to establish a closed circuit. There are challenges after a heart transplant, the most significant of which is the possible rejection of the donor heart. Anytime there is a foreign object in the body, there is a tendency for the body to reject it. Therefore, these patients need to be on drugs to prevent rejection.

Experimental treatments: Some procedures, such as wrapping the heart in a mesh bag to prevent it from enlarging and reducing the left ventricular size by removing segments of the walls, are being evaluated as alternative treatments.

Chapter 29

Blood Clots & Blood Thinners

Blood Clots Can Be Dangerous

A patient of mine was admitted to one of the medical center hospitals with massive swelling in both legs from the groin to the ankles. He had recently traveled from Europe to South America on a nonstop flight while sitting in the plane for 14 hours. He rarely got up from his seat. An ultrasound test confirmed that he had extensive blood clots in his legs obstructing the large veins draining the blood from the legs to the heart that had resulted in the massive swelling of both legs. He was treated with heparin and intravenous blood thinner and later switched to warfarin, an oral blood thinner. He left the hospital with swollen legs.

The abovementioned patient had developed blood clots in the legs, a condition commonly known as deep venous thrombosis or DVT. The blood clots may occasionally travel to the lungs, which occasionally can be fatal.

Where do the blood clots come from? Generally, blood clotting occurs when there is injury to a tissue to prevent further bleeding. However, due to various reasons, the blood clot may develop within the cardiovascular system, which can cause problems. The blood clot could develop in the leg veins or the pelvic veins. From there, they could travel to the lungs. The clots could also develop in the heart chambers and migrate into the circulation, thus blocking an artery in the brain, gut or legs, causing acute and sometimes serious symptoms such as stroke or compromised circulation in the legs (ischemic legs).

Why do people develop blood clots? The blood clotting mechanism can be harmfully affected by various conditions that can predispose a person to develop clots within the veins or arteries. Prolonged rest predisposes people to develop clots, especially in the legs. This can happen in people who sit for a long time where their circulation is cut off or in hospitalized patients who are bedridden and unable to move after surgery, broken bones, or other conditions.

Other conditions that predispose to blood clot formation in the veins are smoking, obesity, minor injuries, hormone contraceptives, and cancer. Irregular heart rhythm such as atrial fibrillation is a frequent cause of clot formation in the heart chambers. That clot can lodge in a brain blood vessel and result in stroke or block an artery in the leg, severely reducing circulation, which can lead to blue toes.

Certain congenital diseases also can alter the blood clotting processes and cause clot formation. These conditions need intensive testing to confirm their diagnosis.

What are the dangers of blood clots? The Blood clots anywhere inside the body could be dangerous and could lead to a variety of complications.

Thrombophlebitis: It is a condition when clots in the calf veins get inflamed and cause swelling, redness, calf pain and tenderness. It can be diagnosed by an ultrasound, which can detect the presence of blood clots in the leg veins. The treatment usually involves bed rest, blood thinners such as heparin for acute treatment and warfarin for 3 to 6 months. The same treatment applies to people with clots in the legs without inflammation. If left untreated, the clots could get bigger and bigger, block the flow of blood through the veins, and increase fluid retention in the legs, leading to poor circulation. The valves within the veins may get damaged, leading to chronic leg swelling.

Pulmonary embolism: It occurs when the clots in the legs or pelvis migrate to the right side of the heart and lodge in the pulmonary veins, resulting in pulmonary embolism, which may become a life-threatening condition. These patients may experience sudden onset of chest pain and shortness of breath. These symptoms may also mimic a heart attack. Time is of the essence in diagnosing this condition. Measurement of blood gases and chest computerized tomography (CT) can help us in establishing the diagnosis of this condition. Initially, these patients are treated with heparin, enoxaparin, or other blood thinners. Later they are maintained on warfarin pills. They need to be on warfarin for 6 to 12 months depending on the extent of the blood clots.

Stroke: Blood clots in the left side of the heart could travel via the arteries and block a tiny artery in the brain, causing a stroke. Bleeding inside the brain also could cause a similar stroke. Therefore, an accurate diagnosis is very important, as the treatment for a blood clot could be different from the treatment for a stroke resulting from bleeding. If a person has a clot, it is treated with standard blood thinners, while patients with bleeding should not receive any blood thinners. The diagnosis of stroke is usually established with the help of a head CT. People diagnosed as having stroke related to a blood clot respond well to clot buster medicine such as tissue plasminogen activator, which dissolves the clot.

Ischemic leg: Sometimes a blood clot in the heart can travel to the legs and cause a blue leg, resulting from total blockage. There will be no pulse beyond the blockage. This is usually a bedside diagnosis. It can also be confirmed with ultrasound and CT angiogram (CTA). The leg may be pale and cold. It is a surgical emergency. The clot has to be removed and then the patient started on blood thinners.

Intestinal ischemia: When blood clots from the heart block one of the small branches in the arteries supplying the intestines, it results in gangrene. This usually happens in patients with multiple medical problems in a hospital setting. It is usually diagnosed by an abdominal CT. The treatment is surgical intervention. Using blood thinners in these complicated patients could be challenging. We have to weigh the advantages versus the risks of further blockages from blood clots.

Heart valves: People with artificial heart valves are also at risk of developing blood clots on the valves. So, these patients are generally maintained on blood thinners lifelong, unless they receive a tissue valve, which has a lesser tendency to bleed. They also need monitoring of their blood to determine the effect of the blood thinners.

Coronary stents: Like heart valves, coronary stents are foreign objects. A coronary stent is a very thin, hallow tube placed in the heart blood vessels, after dilating the coronary arteries. Stents have a tendency to activate the clotting mechanism. Therefore, all coronary stent patients are placed on blood thinners after a stent placement.

What is a blood thinner? A blood thinner blocks various steps in the blood clotting process and increases the time it takes for the blood to form a clot. By prolonging the blood clotting time, the blood thinner prevents new blood clot formation. Aspirin is a weak blood thinner. Plavix is another pill that prevents blood clot formation after coronary stent placement.

In an emergency setting in the hospital, patients receive heparin or enoxaparin as the initial blood thinner. Later, they are placed on warfarin, which is an oral blood thinner. All blood thinners have a tendency to make the blood too thin, to the point where that patient can bleed internally. We have come across people who have bled in the belly or brain because of too thin blood. So, we have to measure the blood thinning effect and keep it between 2.0 to 2.5 times the normal level for people with venous blood clots and between 2.5 to 3.0 for people with heart valves. We also use the international normalized ratio (INR) to measure the blood thinning. The INR tells how a patient is responding to a given blood thinner, and can be measurements in doctors' offices.

How to prevent blood clots? Prevention of blood clots is a major health initiative undertaken in the hospitals. Patients are mobilized early, started on blood thinners such as enoxaparin for prevention, engaged in physical therapy to increase activity, and encouraged to use elastic stockings for the legs. People who are on a plane for long hours or those who are bedridden at home can use similar techniques. Those who travel long distance should exercise their legs every few hours at the ankle and knee joints and move around every few hours to prevent blood clot formation.

Blood Thinners: A Double-Edged Sword

Recently, Josephine, a 78-year-old lady with a critical narrowing of her aortic valve, had her aortic valve replaced with an artificial mechanical valve. She needed a blood thinner to keep her valve from clogging up and constant monitoring of her blood to prevent severe bleeding that might result from too much blood thinner. She does not know the difference between a 5 mg blood thinner and a 10 mg blood thinner. To her they both are the same — a pill!

This patient's story is real and accents the gravity of the situation and what we as physicians need to do and what you as a patient need to understand regarding blood thinners. We will explore what blood thinners are, why people need blood thinners, the types of blood thinners, and the dangers associated with them.

Blood clotting mechanism: Whenever you get a cut, the body has a clotting mechanism to prevent you from bleeding too much. It involves a complex series of chemical reactions that is initiated by tissue injury or a foreign object in the body. In the final analysis, the platelets stick together in a mesh of protein called fibrin that is created during the clotting mechanism. It is like a plug for a leaky pot. However, when a clot develops within a vein, in the lungs, in the heart after valve replacement, or after stent placement, it can be dangerous. In order to prevent this complication, we prescribe blood thinners such as warfarin, aspirin, or Plavix.

Blood thinners serve an essential lifesaving role in most patients with heart valves, blood clots in the legs, veins or lungs, or in those patients who have irregular heart rhythms, such as atrial flutter or fibrillation, among others. In exceptional cases, they may lead to bleeding inside the brain or belly that may prove fatal. Therefore, people who are on blood thinners such as warfarin need constant monitoring of the effect of the blood thinner to assure the blood is not too thin. The word "thinner" is a figurative word used to describe how long it takes for the blood to clot, rather than how thin or thick the blood actually is.

Types of Blood Thinners

Aspirin: Aspirin is a weak blood thinner. It irreversibly binds to the platelets, thus preventing the platelets from sticking to one another. Its action lasts for the lifespan of the platelets. That means, for the body to restore its normal clotting status, it has to replace most of the platelets with new platelets, which may take from 4 to 5 days. Hence, you may hear from your dentist or surgeon to stop taking aspirin 5 days before a major procedure. However, we generally do not recommend people stopping aspirin before cardiac surgery. It takes between 40 and 80 mg of aspirin to achieve the blood thinning effect. It is not useful in patients with blood clots in the veins or lungs. It should be used with caution in patients with a brain hemorrhage or bleeding ulcer. It is very helpful in patients with heart disease. Be aware of aspirin hidden in combination with many cold remedies.

Plavix: It is the most often prescribed blood thinner following coronary stent placement. It is a much stronger blood thinner compared with aspirin. A full dose of Plavix can block anywhere from 50% to 85% of the platelet activity. Just like that of aspirin, the effect of Plavix lasts for the duration of the platelet's life. So patients may have to be off Plavix for 4 to 5 days before any major surgery. However, in an emergency, the surgeon may perform the surgery with a fresh platelet transfusion to prevent bleeding. Abrupt stopping of Plavix without medical supervision could lead to a fresh clot formation that may lead to a heart attack. Therefore, people on Plavix should consult their physician before discontinuing the medicine.

Persantine: It is another weak blood thinner, which is sometimes used in combination with aspirin in patients with mini-strokes (medically known as transient ischemic attacks).

Warfarin: Warfarin (Coumadin) is the Cadillac of all the blood thinners. And, by the same token, it is also the most dangerous if used indiscriminately. It does not break down an existing clot. It simply prevents formation of new clots, while the body's natural mechanisms dissolve the old clot over time. It can prolong the bleeding time by two to ten times normal. Since its effects are very unpredictable, it requires constant monitoring of blood to assure the time it takes to clot is maintained between 2.5 to 3.5 times normal. Nowadays, patients can use portable machines to monitor prothrombin time (PT) and INR to adjust their warfarin dosages with their physician's guidance. Warfarin comes in color-coded tablets, based on dosages. Generally, it is taken once a day in the evening. Never double the dose if you missed the pill one day. Nonsteroidal anti-inflammatory agents (NSAIDs) such as Motrin may make the blood too thin.

In a hospital setting, we use intravenous heparin or subcutaneous enoxaparin in cardiac and surgical patients to prevent acute blood clot formation.

Bleeding problems: There is always a danger of bleeding with all blood thinners. It is most serious with warfarin. Certain foods such as green leafy vegetables like spinach, broccoli, and turnip greens have vitamin K, which may interfere with the warfarin effect. In other words, you may not achieve the desired blood thinning level, and you may have to increase the warfarin dosage to get the needed effect. The following week, when you do not eat those vegetables, your blood may be too thin and may pose a bleeding risk. Some herbs or medicines may increase or decrease blood thinning effect.

Therefore, a very delicate balance has to be established between acceptable blood thinning and the risk of bleeding. If you are on warfarin, maintain a record of blood test results that you get from your portable machines. You also need to avoid foods such as green leafy vegetables that can alter those results. You should also avoid cuts from razor blades and heavy exercise that may cause internal trauma and bleeding.

Management of blood thinner is a team effort between the physician and the patient. Enhancing the patient's understanding is indispensable for achieving the maximum benefit from such treatment. Josephine, my patient, is doing better.

Notes:

Chapter 30

Arterial Diseases

Peripheral Arterial Disease

A 53-year-old male was admitted to the hospital for cardiac surgery. He had already had a heart attack and surgery in the legs two years earlier. In addition, he had a history of diabetes for several years, high cholesterol, and heavy smoking for 20-plus years. He had an uneventful heart surgery and went home. His case raises some important questions regarding the generalized nature of atherosclerosis, or blockages in the arteries. The focus of this article is on the arterial blockages in the legs known as peripheral arterial disease, or PAD.

What causes PAD? The arteries in the pelvis and the legs can develop atherosclerosis, leading to narrowing and blockage of the arteries, causing symptoms of decreased circulation. Atherosclerosis involves the deposition of cholesterol and platelets on the inner lining of the arteries, along with overproduction of smooth muscles. The same process occurs in the heart, the brain, the kidneys, and in other internal organs. When the arterial narrowing approaches 70% of its cross-section, patients develop symptoms of ischemia, or reduced circulation.

The major risk factors for coronary artery disease, such as high cholesterol, smoking, high blood pressure and diabetes, also play a significant role in the development of PAD. In fact, people with PAD are twice as likely to have heart disease as those who do not have PAD. Therefore, we routinely check the heart circulation for those going for vascular surgery in the legs. Diabetes, high blood pressure, and high cholesterol levels are all significant risk factors for PAD. Smoking is a major risk factor for PAD, especially in patients with a history of diabetes or hypertension. Even though PAD affects people in their fifties and sixties, it is not unusual to see people in their late twenties and early thirties having PAD if they have a history of diabetes, hypertension and smoking.

What are the symptoms of PAD? Patients with PAD may complain of pain in the leg that gets worse on walking and is relieved by rest. Only 8% to 10% of the people may have this classical intermittent pain on walking (called intermittent claudication). As the degree of arterial narrowing gets worse, patients may experience pain even at rest. Some patients may not have any symptoms at all. Others with critical blockages and very poor circulation may develop ulcers that do not heal or gangrene. There may also be discoloration of the skin.

Some may experience aching, pain, tightness, cramping, and tiredness in the thigh and hip region brought on by exercise and relieved by rest.

The legs may feel cold because of poor circulation. There is loss of hair and healthy skin texture. Other conditions such as arthritis, sciatica, and diabetic neuropathy can produce similar symptoms.

Diagnosis of PAD

Ankle brachial index: A simple Doppler aided blood pressure measurement at the arms and at the ankles help us to diagnose the presence and severity of PAD. This test is known as the ankle-brachial index. If the ankle pressure is less than 50% of the blood pressure at the arm level, it points to severe arterial disease in the leg. However, it does not help us to establish the location and severity of the arterial blockage that is present.

Duplex scan: To determine the exact location and the extent of the disease, we use an ultrasound duplex scan, which can visualize the location and the degree of the blockage. Doppler velocity measurements help us to determine the functional significance of these blockages.

MRA and CTA: Magnetic resonance arteriograms (MRA) and computerized tomography angiograms (CTA) can identify the presence, the extent, and the location of blockages in the arteries above the knee level.

Arteriography: It is a definitive test where we inject dye to visualize the arteries. The advantage to this approach is that we also can dilate the artery with a balloon or a stent at the same time, if one is needed.

PAD Treatment Options

The main purpose here will be to improve the leg circulation, relieve the symptoms, and prevent further worsening of ulcers or gangrene.

Medications: Minor blockages with mild pain can be initially treated with pills (such as Trental) that improve the manner in which the blood travels, increasing the blood flow. Other medicines include aspirin, Plavix, and cholesterol lowering drugs.

Dilatation: Patients with a localized and critical blockage can be managed with a balloon, stent, or both. They must be on Plavix for 6 to 12 weeks. However, if someone has diabetes, long-term Plavix may be beneficial.

Surgery: People with multiple or total blockages that are not easily amenable to stent treatment may be candidates for vascular bypass, which involves an inpatient stay for 4 to 5 days and surgery. These surgeries go by different names such as aorto-femoral and fem-pop, depending on the blockage level.

How can we prevent PAD? Just as risk factor modification for heart disease leads to improved symptoms and survival rates, similar risk factor modifications can help to reduce the symptoms and decrease the rate at which the disease progresses. Early detection of the problem and its complications may prevent ulceration, infection, and gangrene. Absolute smoking cessation is essential to prevent any further worsening of PAD. Exercise also helps to develop collateral or new channels of circulation and thus improve exercise tolerance.

What is the prognosis? Early recognition and aggressive risk factor modifications may prevent leg amputation, help in healing of leg ulcers, and prevent gangrene formation.

Carotid Artery Disease

Mr. Jason, in his mid-sixties, came to my office with weakness on his right side with some speech difficulty that had lasted for less than 24 hours. Considering that he might have had a transient ischemic attack (TIA or mini-stroke), a complete cardiac and neurological workup was done, which revealed that he had critical blockages in both carotid arteries.

When a patient reports with a transient weakness, dizziness, or visual disturbance, we consider situations related to the heart, such as irregular heart rhythms, a blood clot from the heart lodging in the arteries supplying the brain, or low blood pressure. The blockage of the carotid arteries also can decrease brain circulation and cause these symptoms. There is a host of conditions in the brain such as a hemorrhage, arterial blockage, or tumor that can cause similar symptoms.

What is carotid artery disease? The right and left carotid arteries supply blood to the head, face, and brain. They arise from the major blood vessel called the aorta, in the upper part of the chest. They travel in the neck, in front of the vertebrae. Just below the jaw, they divide into the external carotid branch that supplies blood to the face, skin, and scalp. The internal carotid, the more important branch, supplies the front and middle parts of the brain.

When there is a buildup of plaque, just like the type that happens in the heart and in legs, the arterial cross-section is narrowed. Besides the narrowing, there may be plaque rupture that can release tiny specks of plaque, which can block a tiny branch in the brain and cause TIAs.

What are the symptoms of carotid artery disease? The carotid artery blockage by itself does not give any pain or discomfort in the neck. The majority of symptoms are related to the decreased circulation to the brain resulting from the internal carotid artery blockage. A major stroke may be the first symptom of carotid artery disease. The other symptoms may include a TIA or sudden blindness.

What are the signs of carotid artery disease? Since minor blockage itself does not cause any symptoms, the disease may go undetected until the patient has significant arterial blockages. So it is prudent for the primary care physician to look for signs that may signal carotid artery disease. If your physician routinely listens to both sides of the neck, he or she may pick up some noise in the neck. That may be the first indication of a silent carotid artery disease. If there is an audible bruit (a whooshing noise resulting from arterial narrowing), it deserves further evaluation. Not all bruits come from carotid artery blockage. Some heart murmurs could be transmitted to the neck and appear as though they are coming from the carotid arteries. On the other hand, if there is a critical blockage of one of the arteries, we may not hear any noise at all, as the critical narrowing may severely restrict the blood flow.

How do we diagnose carotid artery blockage? Routine examination of the neck, including listening to the carotid arteries, is the first step. Anyone with a history of multiple risk factors such as hypertension, diabetes, high cholesterol, or arterial disease elsewhere needs special attention. Anyone over age 60 years with or without symptoms must undergo a duplex scan study.

A duplex scan looks not only at the cross-sectional of the carotid artery for any plaque buildup, but also enables us to study the changes in the blood flow to determine the significance of any narrowing. This combined information is very valuable.

When a duplex scan detects a significant problem, that finding has to be confirmed by angiography. There are three types of angiograms, namely, carotid MRA, carotid CT angiogram, and carotid arteriogram.

Carotid MRA: This is a useful noninvasive test in determining the degree of blockage. However, the resolution is not as good as the angiogram. Also, there may be some artifacts created by surrounding structures.

Carotid CT angiogram is gaining some popularity since it is a noninvasive test. However, it involves injection of an intravenous dye, which may harm the kidneys in certain patients. Again, the resolution here is not as good as it is with carotid angiograms. However, to rule out a critical blockage, it could be a useful alternative.

A carotid angiogram: This arteriogram is an invasive procedure that involves inserting catheters in the carotid arteries and taking pictures. This is the most definitive test and has the highest resolution.

The other advantage of performing an angiogram is that we can insert a stent in the carotid artery at the same time, if there is a critical blockage.

The carotid artery has to be blocked more than 70% to cause any significant symptoms. However, if there is a plaque rupture, the degree of blockage does not have to be critical to cause symptoms. The plaque material can lodge in one of the smaller branches in the brain and cause a TIA or even a stroke.

Carotid Artery Disease Management

Medical management depends on symptoms related to the carotid artery blockage. If the person has minimal plaque, the only treatment needed might be a daily intake of 81 mg aspirin. Some people with more advanced disease and with other risk factors such as heart disease or diabetes may benefit from a combination of Plavix and aspirin. Occasionally, neurologists prescribe Aggranox, a combination of aspirin and Persantine.

Carotid stenting: In experienced hands, it has shown good short-term results in terms of complications such as TIA or stroke. However, since this procedure is relatively new, the long-term results are still under investigation.

Carotid endarterectomy (CEA): This has been the gold standard for carotid artery blockage treatment for years. The surgeon opens the blocked carotid artery, scoops out the soft fat-like plaque, and expands the artery's size with a cloth (Dacron) graft, then closes the skin. This involves a one-day stay in the hospital. The risk of stroke following surgery is about 2% to 3%. Most patients do well and remain symptom free for years.

Next time you visit your physician, ask your doctor to listen to your neck.

Transient Ischemic Attacks

Did you ever experience weakness, tingling, or numbness on one side of your body that lasted for minutes or hours? Did you ever feel dizzy, lightheaded, or see things floating in your vision? These symptoms could be a sign of a TIA or a mini-stroke.

What is a TIA or mini-stroke? It is a condition where there is a temporary interruption of blood flow to a tiny part of the brain, resulting in any of the abovementioned symptoms, which last for less than 24 hours. The symptoms may last as little as 5 minutes to less than 24 hours. Sometimes, these symptoms may occur several times during a 24-hour period.

In some people, a TIA or a mini-stroke could occur days, weeks, or months before a full-blown stroke develops. Generally, there is no permanent damage to the brain.

It is more common in men who are over 55, who have a family history of stroke, hypertension, smoking, peripheral arterial disease, diabetes, and/or excess alcohol consumption. It may also be seen in younger women who are taking birth control pills.

What causes a TIA or a mini-stroke? The temporary interruption of brain blood flow could result from several causes, which could be related to the heart, the blood vessels supplying the brain, or the status of the brain blood vessels.

A blood clot in the heart can develop with irregular heartbeats, such as atrial fibrillation, or after a heart attack. This tiny clot can travel to the brain and block a tiny arterial branch, causing symptoms that may be localized to the left or the right side of the body. A very rapid and irregular heart rhythm itself can reduce blood supply to the brain and cause dizziness.

Hardening of the inner layer of the aorta is common in older individuals. Tiny specks from the hardened arterial lining can get detached and block a tiny arterial branch in the brain, causing a TIA or a mini-stroke.

There are two sets of arteries—the carotids and the vertebrals—that supply the brain. As people get older, plaques accumulate in the carotid arteries that can cause mini-strokes or even a full-blown stroke with paralysis involving either side of the body.

With advanced age, the arteries in the brain itself can develop plaques, causing mini or major strokes. A brain hemorrhage usually causes permanent damage. People on blood thinners for prevention of blood clots are at an increased risk for bleeding in the brain.

Severe and uncontrolled hypertension can cause spasms of the brain arteries that can cause TIA symptoms.

What are the manifestations of a TIA or a mini-stroke? TIA, as mentioned at the beginning, can present as weakness, numbness, or tingling, involving the face, arms, and legs. These symptoms usually clear within 24 hours. Some patients may experience dizziness or light-headedness. Others may experience confusion, speaking difficulty, problems related to balance, or unsteady gait. Loss of bladder control, unusual movements, double vision, and partial or complete hearing loss are other symptoms of a TIA or a mini-stroke.

What are the diagnostic steps used in a patient with a TIA or a mini-stroke? Since a TIA or a mini-stroke involves the heart, the blood vessels, and the brain, the diagnosis can be very expensive and time-consuming. The process can be frustrating, as we may not find any definite cause in some patients.

A complete history and physical examination are essential. An elevated blood pressure may be the easiest symptom to recognize and treat. Careful examination of the heart could reveal irregular heart rhythm or extra heartbeats. Listening to the carotid arteries in the neck may reveal a bruit, which may suggest blockage in the arteries going to the brain.

An electrocardiogram can reveal any irregular heartbeats, heart enlargement, or the occurrence of a heart attack in the past. A cardiac ultrasound helps us to identify prior heart attacks, heart enlargement, or the presence of any blood clots.

A carotid artery duplex ultrasound scan shows the presence and severity of carotid artery blockage.

CT angiogram of the head and neck helps us to identify carotid artery blockage or any abnormalities of circulation within the brain. CTA involves injection of contrast material, which is associated with a small risk to the kidneys. CT of the brain may reveal old or new stroke and bleeding.

MRI is very useful in detecting the presence of a stroke in the early hours of its development, whereas a CT scan may not pick up such changes. Again, a CT or an MRI could be normal in patients with a TIA or a mini-stroke. MRI angiography is an alternative non-invasive test to look at the blood vessels supplying the brain.

Angiography is the definite way to determine the extent and severity of carotid or vertebral artery blockage. However, it is an invasive procedure that carries a minimal risk. It also involves injecting contrast material.

What is the treatment for a TIA or a mini-stroke? Any person who comes to a physician with TIA symptoms must be treated as though that person has had a stroke, until we establish a proper diagnosis. The treatment depends on the cause. If it is because of a possible blood clot in a heart chamber, a person may be started on a long-term blood thinner such as Coumadin. Patients on Coumadin need close monitoring of the blood thinner effect and adjustment of the dosage, to minimize any bleeding complications.

The other medicines routinely used include antiplatelet agents. These agents prevent platelets from sticking together, thus minimizing the formation of tiny blood clots that block small arterial segments. Aspirin is the most widely used antiplatelet agent. Plavix is a more potent antiplatelet agent that is also used for prevention of clot formation.

A combination of aspirin and dipyridamole (Persantine) called Aggranox is a popular antiplatelet agent among neurologists.

Patients who have significant carotid artery blockage may benefit from carotid endarterectomy surgery. Carotid artery stenting or angioplasty is an alternative. However, the best long-term results are available only with carotid artery surgery.

Good blood pressure control with diet, exercise, and medications could reduce the risk of stroke by 60%. Reduction in cholesterol and smoking cessation could minimize the plaque buildup in the arteries.

What other conditions can mimic similar symptoms? People with migraine headache may have similar symptoms of numbness and tingling, especially in the face. People with seizure or fainting may have similar symptoms. People with very low blood sugar may also experience similar symptoms.

What is the prognosis? The prognosis from a TIA or mini-stroke itself is good. However, patients who develop this condition are at an increased risk for developing a full-blown stroke and therefore need aggressive evaluation and management to prevent any future TIAs or mini-strokes. Nearly 30% of the people with a TIA go on to develop a full stoke within a year. This underscores the importance of addressing the TIA symptoms in a proactive manner.

For more information on TIA or stroke, visit:
- www.americanheart.org/
- www.stroke.org/
- www.ninds.nih.gov,/
- www.strokeassociation.org/

Chapter 31

Innovations in Treatment

Stent Controversy

Since the introduction of coronary angioplasty by Andrea Gruentzig in 1977 for the treatment of coronary artery disease, we have seen monumental technological advances. Today we can reach the most remote and challenging blockages in the coronary arteries and unclog them. We have discovered better methods of delivering the balloons, keeping the arteries open, and preventing the arterial walls from collapsing by putting in coronary stents, thus reducing the incidence of acute coronary blockages following coronary stent placement. We also have newer medicines to prevent clot formation following a coronary intervention, by using potent antiplatelet agents that prevent clot development.

With the introduction of a bare-metal stent (a steel wire mesh), we can prevent the arterial walls from collapsing and worsening the condition. The stent addressed one of the potential problems inherent during coronary interventions. After stent placement, however, we observed that the original atherosclerosis process, or hardening of the arteries from deposition of cholesterol, was replaced by a new problem, namely, proliferation or overgrowth of the smooth muscle cells in response to the stent (a foreign object). This smooth muscle proliferation extending into the interior of the artery had a tendency to cause reblockage of the coronary arteries in 30% to 50% of the patients who received these bare-metal stents, depending on the size and location of the stents.

To treat this new problem, patients had to undergo repeat cardiac catheterization, involving grinding the new tissue with a tiny Roto-Rooter, by a process known as debulking or atherectomy. The other options are using a cutting balloon to compress the tissue overgrowth or using radiation to shrink the tissue overgrowth. Radiation also reduces the smooth muscle reproduction.

To address the smooth muscle proliferation problem, research has focused on anti-tumor drugs that prevent cell duplication. This led to the introduction of stents coated with drugs embedded between two polymer layers. The drug is gradually released locally at the stent site over 6 to 8 weeks, thus preventing the smooth muscle cell overgrowth. This concept, both in theory and practice, seemed like a novel approach, with one exception.

When we perform a balloon angioplasty or insert a bare-metal stent, we damage the inner lining of the arterial wall, namely, the endothelium, which acts as a lubricant besides performing many other functions. Following the insertion of a bare-metal stent, the endothelium regrows over the stent area and restores the normal arterial wall architecture. This smooth endothelial layer also prevented any new blood clot formation.

However, among those patients who received drug-coated stents, there was a tendency for failure of the regrowth of the endothelial layer to cover the drug-coated stents. That exposed the metal to the blood surface and could act as a stimulus for blood clot formation months and years after the stent placement.

More recently, there have been alarming reports in both the medical and the public media about the adverse effects of drug-coated stents months and years after their insertion. As more and more long-term reports have arrived, the alarm seems to be less than was initially perceived when the news reached the public. The latest research reveals the incidence of acute clot formation in patients with drug-coated stents is less than 0.5% per year. Even though the incidence is very small, the complications from such blockage are very serious and startling. It is not very clear when these complications can occur, thus leaving us with uncertainty.

The outcomes of patients receiving drug-coated stents were not worse off than those who received bare-metal stents. Yet, those who received the drug-coated stents had fewer symptoms and a lesser incidence of blockage or repeat interventions.

To address this very vital problem of clot formation, most cardiologists felt that patients who receive drug-coated stents must be on long-term antiplatelet drugs. However, several medical studies have looked at patients who have been on antiplatelet drugs for up to one year from the time of the coronary stent placement. There is no research data available at present regarding whether patients need to be on antiplatelet drugs longer than one year. Most cardiologists recommend that their patients continue with the antiplatelet drugs, if they have had no major problems with the drugs, until we have a better understanding of the problem.

The antiplatelet drugs simply prevent clot formation, but they still do not address the issue inherent with the drug-coated stents — inhibition of the endothelial regeneration.

What is on the horizon? There is continuing research to look at other methods of keeping the arteries from clogging up after an intervention. Some researchers have used biodegradable stents with no metal involved. The polymers that keep the arterial walls from collapsing are dissolved over an 8 to 12 week period. However, being a foreign object, the polymers themselves have a tendency to stimulate the smooth muscle cells, thus bringing back the problem we had with bare-metal stents. These biodegradable stents treated with drugs are more effective in preventing smooth muscle proliferation. Yet, we are back to the same point; they also inhibit the endothelial regeneration, like their predecessors.

In a span of less than 30 years, we have made more progress in the diagnosis and management of heart disease than we have in the past century before the seventies. Every novel concept comes with its own inherent challenges, which takes us to the next level, and one day we may be able to address the issues that are daunting the cardiologists and the researchers alike.

Medical management of coronary artery disease with aggressive cholesterol lowering, diabetes control, weight reduction, and regular exercise has shown very promising results. It should be part of every heart patient's lifestyle or of every person at a potential risk of developing a heart problem. Consult with your cardiologist before stopping a prescribed antiplatelet drug, as there might be an increased tendency toward new clot formation in the first 90 days after stopping the drug.

Stem Cells & Heart Disease

The words "stem cells" generate a very poignant response from people from all walks of life; from President Bush to the pious pulpit pundits. Some believe it is insane to alter human life or the body by such extreme measures. We will explore the concepts behind stem cell research, the myths surrounding stem cells, and the current research in treating heart diseases, and will look at the future of stem cell research in treating human illness.

What are stem cells? After the sperm fertilizes an egg, a single-cell embryo is formed, which contains the genetic information from both parents. From this one cell, the entire human body is developed in nine months. The original cell divides into billions of cells, which go on to form muscle, nerve, skin, heart, or brain tissue. The embryonic cells retain their potential to transform into any body tissue, depending on the demand, and therefore, they are called stem cells.

Where do these stem cells come from? There are two kinds of stem cells. One type is called pluripotent cells; they come from the human embryo or fetal tissue and can transform into any type of cell in the body. The other type is adult stem cells, which come from adult body parts such as the bone marrow, fat, or heart.

How do stem cells work? The bone marrow, for example, has a type of stem cell (primitive mononuclear cell) that continually produces cells. They continually produce various kinds of red and white blood cells, depending on the need. If someone develops an infection, these stem cells turn up the production of white blood cells to fight the infection. This natural stimulation of cell formation on demand is the basis of implanting the stem cells, for example, in the heart muscle region to stimulate the heart muscle fibers instead of the red or white blood cells. The exact mechanism by which it replicates the heart muscle is not clearly understood. It may replicate the tissue that surrounds it, or it may release hormones that may assist in replicating the tissue.

The same stem cells have been used in various parts of the body to regenerate skin, muscle, and fingers, among other types of tissues that were inconceivable just a few years ago.

What are the concerns? It is a common perception that we have to sacrifice human embryos to harvest the stem cells. Those embryos could have developed into living beings. Therefore, many people believe using embryos is unethical or immoral. It is a legitimate concern. However, most of the stem cells used in cardiac research come from the bone marrow. Stem cells also come from the placentas that are generally discarded after a baby's delivery. Most of the embryonic cells come from eggs fertilized outside the body in test tubes that were not used for the intended purpose of artificial conception. They would go to waste. These embryonic cells are more capable of turning into any type of cell, compared with the adult stem cells which have limitations in their ability to produce different forms of tissue. Therefore, embryonic cells could be used to treat a debilitating disease that is not amenable to any other presently available medical treatments. But others argue the next step would be to use these embryonic stem cells to clone humans.

Therefore, public education becomes a moral obligation and an essential part of any novel research, especially when it involves human life, born or not yet born.

Can stem cells replace damaged heart muscle fibers? When a coronary artery is blocked totally, there is damage to the heart muscle. Generally, patients with this problem undergo cardiac catheterization, where the blockage is opened and a stent placed to prevent abrupt re-blockage. Researchers at the Texas Heart Institute in Houston have used specialized catheters to inject stem cells directly in the proximity of the damaged heart muscle, with the hope of regenerating new heart muscle fibers to improve the overall heart function. The patients receive these stem cells 7 to 10 days after their heart attack. Some centers have injected the stem cells into a coronary artery supplying the damaged heart region. Interestingly, the stem cells not only produce new heart muscle fibers, but also blood vessels, veins, and connective tissue.

If you enroll in such research, it may cost you nothing. Compare that to the $30,000 to $40,000 if you were to travel abroad to get similar treatment.

Although these advances are at the dawn of stem cell research, they appear promising in treating patients with heart attack and severe heart failure.

Can stem cells help patients with heart failure? Patients with heart failure have dilated weak heart muscle with non-contracting fibrous tissue, leading to reduced pumping efficiency of the heart. When these patients receive stem cells, there is an overall improvement in the heart pumping function, with more areas moving compared with before the treatment, and improvement in exercise capacity.

Can stem cells help poor arterial circulation in the legs? People with peripheral arterial disease have severe multiple blockages in the leg arteries, leading to poor circulation, pain, ulceration, and in worst cases, gangrene, calling for amputation. Researchers at the Texas Heart Institute have shown improvement in the formation of new channels of circulation (collateral circulation) in the legs, by directly injecting stem cells several times into the leg calf muscles. Patients get some relief of symptoms and can walk an increased distance.

What is the future for stem cells? Stem cell research has shown promising results in treating conditions such as Parkinson's disease, Alzheimer's, diabetes, arthritis, spinal cord injuries, burns, and others. With further improvements in obtaining and pretreating the cells, the stem cells' effectiveness may improve. With the government commitment to stem cell research and increased funding, more and more data should be coming in the future.

New Indicators for Heart Disease

Heart disease is the number one cause of overall disability and death in the United States. Despite significant advances in understanding cardiac risk factors and the diagnosis and management of cardiovascular diseases, it is perplexing to note that more than 40% of the people who have heart attacks have normal cholesterol levels. This has energized researchers to look at indicators beyond the normal risk factors, to identify those people who may be at an increased risk of developing future cardiovascular events and take measures to reduce those events.

An observational study involving more than 85,000 nurses showed that those who had elevated levels of C-reactive protein (CRP), a marker for low-level inflammation, had a higher incidence of vascular events compared with those with normal CRP levels.

Several small-scale studies have shown that those who were getting statins (drugs to lower high LDL cholesterol levels) benefited more when they had elevated CRP levels in comparison to those who had normal CRP levels.

A landmark study reported at the American Heart Association annual meeting in 2009 shed some light on a new indicator. This might help us identify a population with minimal traditional risk factors such as hypertension, diabetes, and high cholesterol who may be at an increased risk for developing heart disease.

This study, called JUPITER (acronym for Justification for the Use of statins in Prevention and Intervention Trial Evaluating Rosuvastatin), involved 17,802 patients. It was based on the hypothesis that people with elevated levels of CRP may be at an increased risk of developing cardiovascular disease. C-reactive protein can readily be measured in any laboratory.

The study selected 17,802 people with no history of hypertension or diabetes and normal LDL cholesterol levels. They were included in the study because they had a CRP level above 2.0 mg/L. The average CRP in the treated group was 4.2 mg/L in comparison to 4.3 mg/L in the placebo or control group. It also excluded people with known history of heart disease, or those who were already on statins. The study population included a wide spectrum of people, including Caucasians, women, African-Americans, Hispanics, and others.

Half the people in the group (8901) received 20 mg rosuvastatin (cholesterol lowering drug) while the other half received a placebo. Four years into the research, the study was prematurely terminated in March 2008 because of overwhelmingly positive results in favor of the rosuvastatin treated group.

In the rosuvastatin treated group, there was a 50% reduction in the LDL cholesterol, a 4% increase in the HDL cholesterol, a 17% decrease in the triglycerides, and a 37% decrease in the CRP levels. The LDL level was less than 50 mg/dL in the treatment group.

At the end of four years, cardiovascular endpoints such as heart attack, stroke, unstable angina (chest pain), bypass surgery, stent placement, and cardiovascular related deaths were monitored. In the placebo group, 251 out of the 8901 people experienced the above-mentioned event(s), while in the rosuvastatin treated group, there were only 142 such incidences. Overall, the rosuvastatin treated group experienced a 44% reduction in these endpoints. These benefits were noted across the board in men, women, smokers, non-smokers, people less than 65 and people more than 65. Similar benefits were seen in people with or without hypertension, people with or without a family history of heart disease, and people who were normal weight or overweight. There was a 20% reduction in all causes of death in the treated group. There was also a 47% reduction in the rates of hospitalization or revascularization (bypass surgery or new stent placement) in the rosuvastatin group over a two year period.

Most of the side effects, such as muscle weakness or other muscle problems, and cancer incidence were similar in both groups. There was a slight increase in the incidence of diabetes; 3% in the treated group in comparison to 2.4% in the placebo group. Overall, the drug was well tolerated by the group.

Another study (AFCAPS/TEXCAPS) studied 5740 men and women with average cholesterol levels, low HDL, and no cardiovascular diseases who received lovastatin or placebo. The treatment group showed a 37% reduction in the risk of first coronary events.

Here also, the study noted an increased incidence of cardiac events in those who had higher CRP levels. Those who had higher levels of CRP but low levels of LDL cholesterol had cardiac events equal to those who had higher LDL levels, suggesting that high levels of CRP were as risky as the elevated levels of LDL in predicting future cardiac events. The treated group also had a 15% reduction in the CRP levels.

Another inflammatory marker that has gained attention is lipoprotein-associated phospholipase A2 (Lp-PLA2). It has been shown to recognize the presence or formation of rupture-prone plaque. Lifestyle modification, including diet and exercise along with lipid lowering agents, can be effective in lowering the Lp-PLA2.

WASCOPS (West of Scotland Coronary Prevention Study Group), reported in 1995, was an earlier study that looked at using the cholesterol lowering drug pravastatin in reducing cardiovascular events. This study involved 6595 men without a history of heart attack. At the end of five years, the combined cardiovascular events were 5.5% in the treatment group compared with 7.9% in the placebo group.

There were two additional points of information derived from this study that are noteworthy. After the study was completed, the same people were followed for the next five years. Interestingly, the group that had received the pravastatin continued to show lower cardiovascular events compared with those who received placebo during the study, despite many in the treatment group no longer taking the drug. One explanation was that by reducing the LDL levels, they were perhaps able to stabilize the plaque, which provided a long-term benefit even after the drug was discontinued. The second point was related to the CRP. When the researchers went back and looked at the CRP data they had gathered from the study population, they found that a combination of elevated Lp-PLA2, cholesterol, and high CRP levels correlated highly with increased future cardiovascular events.

Another area of interest in detecting a vulnerable plaque that is likely to rupture and cause a heart attack is in the imaging area. The CT scanners available today can identify the coronary arteries and plaque buildup within those arteries. However, the present-day CT scanners cannot differentiate the plaques in various stages of formation. We can detect a calcium buildup within a plaque. However, we are not yet able to tell the difference between a stable and an unstable plaque. It is the unstable plaque that is of a greater concern, because a thin plaque surface can rupture and leading to clot formation that can eventually block the coronary arteries, resulting in a heart attack.

These studies have enabled us to take a step further in identifying people who might be at risk of developing cardiovascular problems and trying to reduce such events before they have an effect on the patients. This will change the way we look at existing risk factors while considering the new identifiers when we see patients either for the first time or after a negative cardiac workup. The novel approach in heart disease risk treatment is to use statins if someone has elevated LDL cholesterol, diabetes, or CRP of greater than 2.0 mg/L, along with diet, weight control, and exercise.

Conclusion

In conclusion, Heart Healthy Living is a life transforming phenomenon. Many people who have had a heart attack or heart surgery, embrace this concept. Why not live a Heart Healthy Lifestyle now, so your family and you can enjoy years of happiness and joy.

Even if this book has provided you with one tip that has made a positive difference in your life, it has been worth your time and my time.

Now, could you please make a difference in the life of a family member or a friend by recommending this book to that person.

You can also look for this book in an eBook or iPad format in the near future.

If you have any comments, questions, or suggestions for the future, please let me know.

If you want me to make a presentation before your group, please contact me at nikam@windstream.net.

Nik

Dr. Nikam's Heart Healthy Lifestyle Chart

1	Reduce your calorie intake to less than _____/day (1200 to 1800) for weight loss.
2	Reduce carbohydrate intake to 200 to 800 calories, 50 to 200 grams/day for weight loss.
3	Keep fat intake to less than 20% to 30% of total calories (240 to 540 calories), or 26 to 60 grams/day.
4	Minimize intake of solid fats, sweets, butter, and lard.
5	Consume less than 15% to 25% of total calories (180 to 300) as protein, or 45 to 100 grams/day.
6	Look for skim milk instead of regular, 2% or 1% milk.
7	Select fiber-rich products: Fiber One, All-Bran, Raisin Bran, or Kashi.
8	Take 1 tbsp of Bene-fiber with 2 to 3 glasses of water (lowers cholesterol level).
9	Consider a glass (3.5 oz) of red wine per day (it is high in antioxidants, reduces heart-disease risk).
10	Consume 2 to 3 fish oil capsules twice a day (omega-3s reduce heart disease risk).
11	Take one flaxseed oil capsule twice daily (omega-3s reduce heart disease risk).
12	Consider 500 mg of niacin 1 to 3 times per day (lowers cholesterol level).
13	Exercise: Walk for 30 to 45 minutes per day or jog for 15 to 20 minutes per day. Burn at least 300 calories daily with aerobic exercise.
14	Restrict meats to less than 8 oz/day. Select chicken, turkey, lean meat, beans, peas, or veggie patties.
15	Consume fish such as salmon, mackerel, tuna, or sardines 2 to 3 times per week (omega-3s reduce heart disease risk).
16	Select salads with low-calorie dressings every day.
17	Watch a comedy channel: Get a sense of humor; it's good for the soul and nerves.
18	Downsize your belt. Never upsize your belt. Just say no.
19	Drink at least 8 glasses of water a day.
20	Take one Centrum A to Z daily.
21	Consider one aspirin tablet per day (81 or 325 mg).

Low Glycemic Index Foods--Part-1

Foods	QNT	Carb-g	GI
All-Bran breakfast cereal	1/2 cup	15	30
Apple, 1 medium	4 oz.	15	38
Basmati rice, white, boiled	1 cup	38	58
Black-eyed peas, canned	2/3 cup	17	42
Bun, hamburger	1.5 oz.	22	61
Carrots, mean of four studies, raw	1 med.	6	47
Chickpeas, canned	2/3 cup	22	42
Coca-Cola soft drink	8 oz.	26	53
Cucumber	3/4 cup	0	0
Fructose, pure	1 Tbsp	10	19
Gluten-free split pea and soy pasta shells	1 1/2 cups	31	29
Grapefruit, raw, medium	1/2	11	25
Green peas	1/3 cup	7	48
Hot cereal, unflavored	1.2 oz. dry	19	25
Ice cream, low-fat vanilla "light"	1/2 cup	9	50
Kidney beans	3/4 cup	18	46
Lentils, green, boiled	3/4 cup	17	30
Lima beans, baby, frozen,	3/4 cup	30	32
Macaroni, cooked	1 1/4 cups	48	47
Milk, skim	8 oz.	13	32
Mousse, chocolate, 2% fat	1.75 oz.	11	31
Mousse, mango, 1.8% fat	1.75 oz.	11	33
Mousse, mixed berry, 2.2% fat	1.75 oz.	10	36
Mousse, strawberry, 2.3% fat	1.75 oz.	10	32
Multi-grain 9-grain bread	1 oz.	14	43
Noodles, mung bean, dried, boiled	1 1/2 cup	45	39
Oatmeal	1 cup	21	42
Orange, medium	4 oz.	11	42
Peach, large	4 oz.	11	42
Peanuts, roasted, salted	1.75 oz.	6	14
Pear, raw	4 oz.	11	38

Carbohydrates=4, proteins=4, fats=9, and alcohol=7 calories,
Carb= carbohydrates, g=grams, GI=Glycemic Index

Low Glycemic Index Foods--Cont.

Foot item	QNT	Carb-g	GI
Pinto beans, dried, boiled	3/4 cup	26	39
Plums, raw	2 med	12	39
Ravioli, wheat flour, meat filled, boiled	6.5 oz.	38	39
Rice, brown, steamed	1 cup	33	50
Rice noodles, freshly made, boiled	1 1/2 cups	39	40
Rye bread	1 oz.	14	58
Soybeans, dried, boiled	1 cup	6	20
Spaghetti, white, boiled 5 min.	1 1/2 cups	48	38
Spaghetti, whole wheat, boiled 5 min.	1 1/2 cups	44	32
Split pea and soy pasta shells, gluten-free	1 1/2 cups	31	29
Split peas, yellow, boiled 20 min.	3/4 cup	19	32
Super Supreme pizza, thin and crispy	1 slice	22	30
Tapioca, boiled with milk	3/4 cup	18	81
100% whole grain bread	1 oz.	13	51
Yogurt, low-fat, fruit, with artificial sweetener	8 oz.	15	14
Apple juice, pure, clear, unsweetened	250 ml	30	44
Smoothie, spy, banana	250 ml	22	30
White bread +15 g psyllium fiber	30 g	17	41
All-Bran (Kellogg's)	30 g	23	38
Hot cereal, apple and cinnamon	30 g	22	37
Rice, basmati, boiled	1 cup	38	58
Rice, brown, steamed	1 cup	33	50
Yogurt, type	200 ml	9	36
Low-fat, fruit, aspartame, Ski	200 g	13	14
Soy milk	250 ml	17	44
Apple	Medium	16	40

Carbohydrates=4, proteins=4, fats=9, and alcohol=7 calories

High Glycemic Index Foods: Part-1

Foods	QNT	Carb-g	GI
Broken rice, white, cooked in rice cooker	1 cup	43	86
Cantaloupe, raw	4 oz.	6	65
Clif bar (cookies & cream)	2.4 oz.	34	101
Corn Flakes, Honey Crunch breakfast cereal	1 cup	24	72
Corn Pops breakfast cereal	1 cup	26	80
Crispix breakfast cereal	1 cup	25	87
Desiree potato, peeled, boiled 35 min.	5 oz.	17	101
Doughnut, cake type	1.75 oz.	23	76
English muffin	1 oz.	14	77
French baguette, white, plain	1 oz.	15	95
French fries, frozen, reheated in microwave	30 pcs.	29	75
Gatorade sport drink (orange)	8 oz.	15	80
Glucose tablets	3 pcs.	15	102
Gluten-free white bread, sliced	1 oz.	13	79
Glutinous rice, white, cooked in rice cooker	2/3 cup	48	92
Instant potato, prepared	3/4 cup	20	85
Instant rice, white, cooked 6 min.	3/4 cup	42	87
Jasmine rice, white, cooked in rice cooker	1 cup	42	109
New potato, unpeeled and boiled 20 min	5 oz.	21	78
Pancakes, prepared from mix	4" 2	58	67
Potato, baked	5 oz.	30	85
Pretzels, oven-baked	1 oz.	20	83
Rice, parboiled	1 cup	36	72
Rice Krispies breakfast cereal	1 1/4 cups	26	87
Rice pasta, brown, boiled 16 min.	1 1/2 cups	38	92
Roll-ups processed fruit snacks	1 oz.	25	99
Soda crackers, Premium	5	17	74
Total breakfast cereal	3/4 cup	22	76
Waffles	1	13	76
Watermelon, raw	4 oz.	6	72

Carbohydrates=4, proteins=4, fats=9, and alcohol=7 calories.

High Glycemic Index Foods--Cont.

Foods	QNT	Carb-g	GI
White bread	1 oz.	14	70
Whole-wheat bread, wheat flour	1 oz.	12	77
Doughnut, cake type	Medium	23	76
Corn muffin, low-amylose	57 g	29	102
Pancakes, buckwheat, gluten-free, made from packet mix	77 g	22	102
Scones, plain (packet mix)	25 g	9	92
Coca-Cola soft drink	250 ml	26	63
White flour	30 g	14	70
Lebanese bread, white	30 g	16	75
Middle Eastern flatbread	30 g	16	97
Wheat flour flatbread	30 g	16	66
Amaranth-wheat composite flour flatbread	30 g	15	76
Corn Flakes (Kellogg's)	30 g	26	92
Cream of Wheat	250 g	26	66
Amaranth, popped, with milk	30 g	22	97
Rice, long grain, parboiled, cooked 20 min.	1 cup	37	75
Jasmine rice	1 cup	42	109
Banana, ripe (all yellow)	Medium	25	51
Dates, dried	60 g	40	103

Carbohydrates = 4, proteins = 4, fats = 9, and alcohol calories.

Notes:

Notes: